Dementia- A Way Ahead

Written by

Jagdish Prasad Yadav

(Senior Occupational Therapist)

Book Description

This book was created to encourage you to learn about Dementia in detail and how to prevent it. Even if dealing with Dementia or preventing it may seem insurmountable, think of it as a journey of helping your loved ones in difficult times.

During my career as an occupational therapist, I have come across various cases of dementia. Thereby, I understand the difficulties that the patient and their families face. My experience and knowledge have enabled me to make this complete guide for you.

It is ideal for someone experiencing dementia or for their family. From understanding the diagnosis, getting assessments done, and helping them in a wide variety of ways- I have got everything covered in this book for you.

As you read through the book, you will find it informative and easy to understand. The incremental information and guidance will help you prevent dementia, diagnose it at the right time, and manage it accordingly.

So, let's get started!

Disclaimer

Content

(A) Dementia Introduction

What is Dementia?

When the same eyes that have once looked at you with adoration haze into a struggle for recognition, it does a little more than break your heart.

Dementia is indicative of diseases affecting parts of the brain, generally used for memory, learning, language, and the ability to carry out day-to-day tasks. It slowly affects mental functioning, like planning, judgment, and abstract thinking and creates psychiatric disorders such as agitation, delusions, and depression.

Since it is a pathological process in the brain that reduces the quality of life, dementia patients gradually require more and more help. According to the WHO, Dementia affects older people more often. Every year almost 10 million new cases are registered, and the estimated population is 60 and over. However, during my career as an occupational therapist, I have noticed that many people confuse Dementia with forgetfulness during ageing, though the symptoms are quite different.

Technically it creates difficulties with the following:

Reasoning,

Emotions,

Judgment,

Memory, and

It is usually associated with difficulties in speaking or writing coherently (or understanding what is said or written), recognizing unfamiliar surroundings, and planning and carrying out multi-step tasks.

Types of Dementia

There are approximately 100 types of Dementia, each having its causes. Some of the most common forms of Dementia are:

Alzheimer's disease

Vascular Dementia

Dementia with Lewy bodies (DLB) and Parkinson's disease dementia (PDD)

Frontotemporal Dementia (FTD)

1. Alzheimer's Disease

The most generic form of dementia, Alzheimer's dementia, predominantly affects the grey matter structures. But, particularly around the brain's outside areas, it will also affect some of the grey matter structures deep inside the brain. So I'm drawing here what we would look at in terms of the hippocampus.

Alzheimer's disease causes excessive and abnormally folded proteins to accumulate in the brain, damaging individual brain cells. Hence, the brain is unable to work like it used to. Moreover, the neurotransmitters (chemical 'messengers') are also affected, disrupting memory, other mental abilities, and communication within the brain.

A combination of factors contributing to the disease's onset and progression include genetic inheritance, age, environmental factors, diet, and overall general health. People with Down Syndrome are also at risk of developing dementia as they grow older. Alzheimer's disease is the most common cause that affects them.

2.Vascular-Dementia

Vascular Dementia is the second most common type of Dementia, caused by narrowing blood vessels in the brain, a series of minor strokes called 'Transient ischemic attacks (TIA),' or a combination of both. It may also result from 'small vessel disease' called 'sub-cortical vascular dementia,' or inswinger's disease), in which blood vessels lying deep in the brain become damaged. This affects the blood supply to the brain cells. The risk factors include heart problems, high blood pressure, high cholesterol, and diabetes. People, in addition, people with vascular Dementia often have difficulty concentrating and communicating.

3. Dementia with Lewy Bodies (DLB) and Parkinson's Disease Dementia(PDD)

Lewy bodies are spherical protein deposits that build up in brain cells, interfere with the chemical 'messengers' in the brain, and disrupt the brain's normal functioning. This affects memory and other mental abilities, like Alzheimer's Disease. Symptoms progress over the years and vary daily. Patients may also suffer physical problems such as stiffness, rigidity, slow movements, and tremors/weakness in the arms and legs. In addition, they may experience visual hallucinations or see things that are not common. Lewy bodies are also found in the brains of people with Parkinson's disease. Therefore, 40% of people with Parkinson's disease may develop dementia. The relationship between DLB and PDD is complicated: it is thought that while the two conditions are part

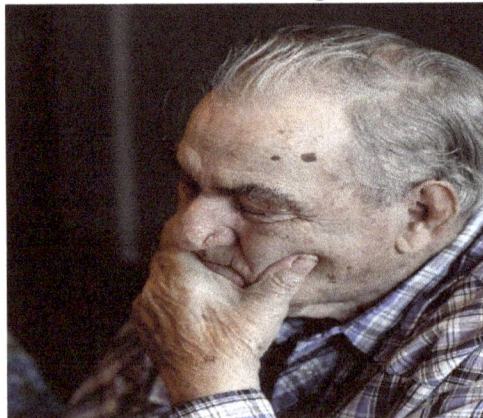

of the same continuum, they produce different signs and symptoms as a result of the further distribution of Lewy bodies in the brain.

4. Frontotemporal Dementia (FTD)

Also known as Picks Disease, Frontotemporal dementia is a rarer form of dementia that affects the brain's front and side. It covers a range of conditions, such as frontal lobe degeneration and Dementia associated with motor neuron disease. It is either hereditary or caused by damage to the brain's frontal or temporal lobe areas. Even though the person's memory may be acceptable, there may be changes in language skills, personality, and behaviour.

5. Other Rare Types

Some less common causes include Huntington's disease, prion diseases, alcohol-related dementias (such as Korsakoff's Syndrome and Creutzfeldt-Jakob disease), HIV, multiple sclerosis, and Dementia resulting from syphilis. Moreover, a link has been suggested between head injury and the later development of Dementia, although this remains controversial

(B) Historical Perspective

Dementia history dates back to 2000 BC when Egyptian psychiatrists first documented the concept. However, it was not until 1797 that the phenomenon was named. Derived from Latin, the word dementia means 'out of one's mind.' A French psychiatrist, Philippe Pinel, first coined the term.

The Oxford Dictionary defines dementia as a severe mental disorder caused by brain disease or injury that affects thinking, remembering, and behaving normally.

During the 18th century, dementia was a term for people with an intellectual deficit. However, by the end of the 19th century, the term was only used for people with cognitive ability loss.

Simultaneously, the term 'senile dementia' was also introduced by Doctor James Cowles Prichard in his book, *A Treatise on Insanity*. The word senile, which means 'old, 'is attached to any insanity in older people. Since one of the most prominent symptoms of dementia is memory loss, it is primarily associated with old age.

Dementia is a broad term used for disorders that affect the brain. Previously, syphilis was considered the common cause of dementia. However, it was only in 1906 that Alzheimer's was identified as the primary culprit.

In 1901, a 51-year-old woman, August D's husband, admitted her to the state asylum in Frankfurt as she was suffering from paranoia, memory loss, aggressive behaviour, speech issues, and hallucinations. Dr Alois Alzheimer followed her case. In 1903, Alois moved to Munich to work with Emil Kraepelin - a well-known psychiatrist.

In 1906, when August D died, her brain was sent to Dr Alois for examination. While presenting the post-mortem report, Dr Alois mentioned August D's cognitive and non-cognitive deficits, highlighting plaques, arteriosclerotic changes, and tangles in her brain. He wrote: "The autopsy reveals, according to Alzheimer's description, changes that represent the most serious form of senile dementia... the Drusen were numerous, and almost one-third of the cortical cells had died off. In their place instead, we found peculiar deeply stained fibrillary bundles that were closely packed to one another and seemed to be remnants of degenerated cell bodies."

The plaques and tangles identified by Dr Alois are the leading causes of Alzheimer's, including the loss of connection between nerve cells. The plaques and tangles are formed due to abnormal deposits of protein. Usually, no symptoms appear during the initial stages of the disease. It is believed that brain damage starts a decade before any cognitive problems surface. The damage begins in the hippocampus, which is responsible for memory. Once neurons start dying, they shrink, and by the final stage, considerable damage is done, which makes the disease irreversible. Major studies and research have been done since Dr Alois's discovery. In 1931, Max Knoll and Ernst Ruska invented the electron microscope. With magnification up to 1 million times, the microscope helped scientists study brain cells with greater depth. In 1983, an entire month was dedicated to Alzheimer's Disease to raise awareness. In 1984, the National Institute of Aging started supporting Alzheimer's disease centres and established a nationwide research network.

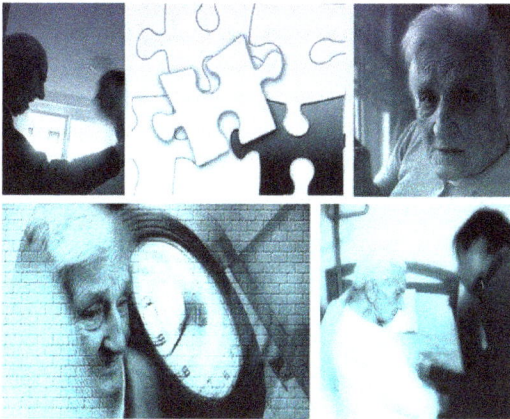

(C) What Are the Early Signs of Dementia?

It is a common fact that dementia patients might not recognise who you are. For example, they may think it's the winter of 2018, even though you tell them it's 2021.

You may cut out a few slices of a rosy apple for them, and they will keep it in their mouth, forgetting to chew and swallow till you remind them, so give them an easy-to-swallow meal like warm soup and mashed bananas.

Your back may feel pain from helping them move around because they may forget to walk; it requires carrying.

As a result, they will be anxious, confused, and irritable.

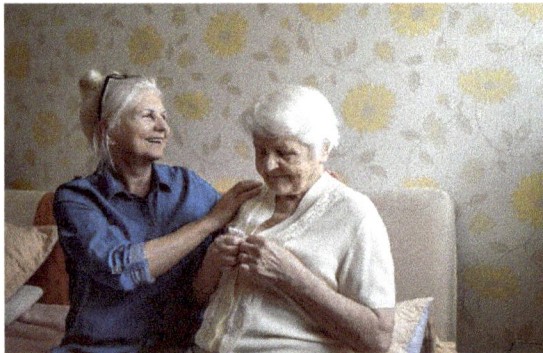

Each person's experience with dementia is unique. Not everyone will experience all the signs and symptoms of their type of dementia. The condition is progressive, and the early signs may be difficult to detect. How the illness progresses varies from person to person. In the beginning, there may be slight memory lapses and altered mood. Later, more apparent problems may develop.

There are vivid descriptions by people with dementia of their own experience of these early-stage symptoms. For example, Malcolm Pointon, a musician with early-onset dementia, wrote in his diary: "Mind in a fog today ... thoughts and actions slipping from my grasp ... kept close to Barbara in the shops ... just didn't want to talk ... head full of cotton wool."

Caretakers have also commented on distressing changes in behaviour: "There was something I said to him, and he went berserk, turned very nasty ... It wasn't like him."

Dementia symptoms vary depending on the cause, but common signs and symptoms include:

1.Cognitive Changes

1. loss, which a spouse usually notices or someone else - Forgetting the names of objects and people.
2. Forgetting where things are and events that have recently occurred.

2. Difficulty in Speech

1) Communicating or finding words.
2) Forgetting phrases or using incorrect words in sentences.

3. Apathy- Needing encouragement to do easy tasks or lacking interest in all interests or hobbies

4. Difficulty in Thinking- Does not understand the alphabet having difficulty with numbers.

5. Difficulty with coordination and motor functions- Putting on clothes in the incorrect order or incorrectly and becoming accident-prone.

6. Confusion and disorientation- Unsure of date, month, where they are, or how to get home.

7. Movements- Pacing restlessly or unsteadily. Agitation.

8. Difficulty with visual and spatial abilities, such as getting lost while driving.

9. Difficulty reasoning and problem-solving

10. Difficulty handling tasks - such as brushing teeth, shaving, dressing, or making a cup of tea difficult

11. Difficulty with planning and organising

Psychological Changes

Personality changes

Depression

Anxiety

Inappropriate behaviour

Paranoia

Agitation

Hallucinations

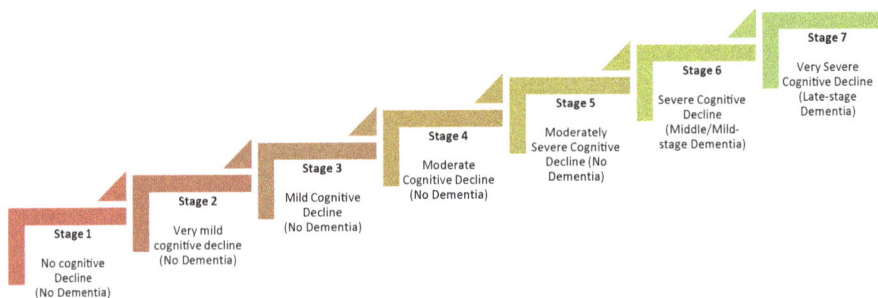

Figure 1: Stages of Dementia

Stages	Signs and Symptoms
Stage 1	In the first stage, the person shows normal function, has no memory loss and is mentally healthy. People with no dementia would be in Stage 1, which is called no cognitive decline (no dementia)
Stage 2	The second stage describes normal forgetfulness associated with ageing, for example, forgetfulness of names and familiar objects. Symptoms are not evident to loved ones or the physician. That is called very mild cognitive decline (no dementia)
Stage 3	The 3rd stage of dementia includes increased forgetfulness, slight difficulty concentrating, decreased work capacity, and an average duration of up to 7 years. In addition, people may need help finding the right words. At this stage, a person's loved ones begin to notice a cognitive decline. It is called mild cognitive decline (no dementia).
Stage 4	This stage includes difficulty concentrating, decreased memory of recent events, and difficulties managing finances or travelling alone to new locations. The average duration is two years. In addition, people have trouble completing complex tasks efficiently or accurately and may be in denial about their symptoms. They may also start withdrawing from family or

	friends because socialisation becomes difficult. At this stage, a physician can detect obvious cognitive problems during patient interviews and exams. It is called moderate cognitive decline (no dementia)
Stage 5	This stage duration holds at least 1.5 years. People in this stage have significant memory deficiencies and need assistance to complete their daily activities (dressing, bathing, and preparing meals). Memory loss is more prominent and may include relevant aspects of current lives. For example, people may need to remember their address or phone number and may not know the time, day, or location. It is called a moderately severe cognitive decline (no dementia).
Stage 6	People in Stage 6 require extensive assistance to carry out daily activities. They start to forget the names of close family members and have little memory of recent events. Many people can remember only some details of their earlier life. They also have difficulty counting down from 10 and finishing tasks. Incontinence (loss of bladder or bowel control) is a problem in this stage. Ability to speak declines. Personality changes, such as delusions (believing something to be true that is not), compulsions (repeating a simple behaviour, such as cleaning), or anxiety and agitation, may occur. Average duration: 2.5 years. It is called severe cognitive decline

	(middle/ mild-stage dementia).
Stage 7	People in this stage have essentially no ability to speak or communicate. Its average duration is 2.5 years. They require assistance with most activities (e.g., using the toilet and eating). They often lose psychomotor skills, for example, the ability to walk. It is called very severe cognitive decline (late-stage dementia).

(D) People at Higher Risks

Researchers have discovered several important factors that affect our risk of developing Dementia. Apart from age and genetics, medical conditions and lifestyle choices are equal contributors. The risk of developing Dementia depends on a combination of all of these.

Factors such as age and genes are passed on through generations; hence we cannot change them. However, other factors, including our lifestyles and how we treat our medical conditions, can be controlled – e.g., by reducing smoking, exercising, eating a good diet, sleeping well, managing stress, etc.

The different risk factors of Dementia become important at various stages in our lives. For example, the 'newness' and 'complexity' of activity drive the production of new connections (synapses) in the brain and contribute toward our 'cognitive reserve.' This is why education at a younger age is protective against the development of dementia. Interestingly, there is a dose-response, meaning the more education you have before year 12, the more protected you are.

Similarly, many studies show that staying in education beyond 16 reduces your risk of dementia later in life. Likewise, stopping smoking probably still lowers your dementia risk. However, why not try not smoking to prevent future risks?

Most of the crucial avoidable risk factors for Dementia, such as type 2 diabetes and high blood pressure, tend to first appear between the ages of about 40 and 64. This is because the changes in the brain that cause Dementia seem to start in middle age. Therefore, mid-life is a critical time to adopt healthy behaviours if you are not already doing so.

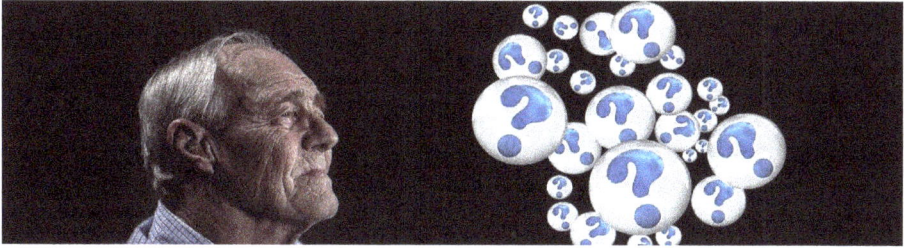

Suppose you have a family history of specific factors that can lead to Dementia or know a loved one who has developed the disease. In that case, it is natural to ask why Dementia occurs. You should read the following factors and consider if you suffer from any of them and which can be controlled.

1. Age

Ageing is the primary cause of Dementia. Even though it is possible to develop the disease earlier, at least 1 in 20 people develop it under 65. Above the age of 65, the risk of developing Alzheimer's disease or Vascular Dementia doubles every five years. This shows that the chances of developing dementia rise significantly older age. It is estimated that Dementia affects one in 14 people over 65 and one in six over 80.

2. Gender

According to research, women are more likely to develop Alzheimer's disease than men. While the reasons are unclear, this is a genuine factor even if we consider the face to live longer on average.

It has been suggested that Alzheimer's disease in women is linked to a lack of estrogen after menopause. For most dementias except Alzheimer's disease, men and women are equally at risk. However, for vascular Dementia, men are slightly at a higher risk than women. This is because they are more prone to stroke and heart diseases, which can cause vascular and mixed Dementia.

15

3.Ethnicity

There is some evidence that people from specific ethnic communities are at higher risk of Dementia than others. For example, South Asian people (from countries such as India and Pakistan) seem to develop Dementia – particularly vascular Dementia – more often than white Europeans. This can be because South Asians are well known to be at a higher risk of stroke, diabetes, and heart disease.

Similarly, people of African or African-Caribbean origin seem to develop Dementia more often. This is because they are known to be more prone to strokes and diabetes. This variation can be because of genes, diet, exercise, and smoking differences.

4. Family History/Genetics

As we all know, the genes we inherit from our parents can affect whether or not we will develop certain diseases. Having a close relative (parent or sibling) with Dementia increases your chances of developing the disease. This varies slightly as compared to someone with no family history. However, this doesn't eliminate the chances of you developing Dementia.

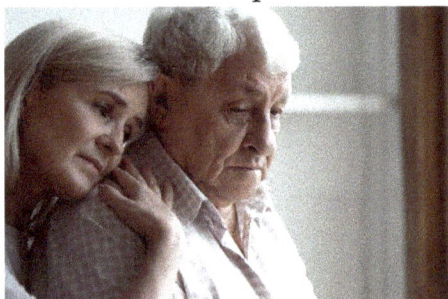

In families where Dementia has been running for generations, there is an evident pattern of inheritance of Dementia from one generation to the other. For example, if a person has a faulty gene, then each of their children has a 50 per cent chance of inheriting it and developing Dementia.

5. Medical Conditions and Diseases

- High blood pressure/ Cardiovascular risk factors in midlife: cerebrovascular lesions, chronic heart failure, low pulse pressure & low diastolic pressure
- High Cholesterol (Serum) in midlife: Saturated fats & Homocysteine
- Diabetes & Pre-diabetes/Impaired Glucose Metabolism in midlife or later life
- Excessive weight and obesity in midlife

6. Depression or Psychological Distress

The other critical, confusing diagnosis is depression because depression in the elderly can look precisely like dementia. So, it takes careful differential diagnosis to separate whether the person is suffering from dementia or depression. The other thing is that many people with dementia in the earlier stages become depressed, and we have to recognise it.

Therefore, it is unclear whether depression is a risk factor that causes Dementia, and the answer probably varies with age. However, there is some evidence that depression in middle age does lead to higher dementia risk in older age. Whereas depression in later life, i.e., when a person is 60's or older, may be an early symptom of Dementia rather than a risk factor for it.

7.Lifestyle-Factors

According to research, there is adequate evidence that our lifestyle choices affect our risk of developing Dementia. This is particularly true of activities linked to cardiovascular health. In addition, studies of large groups show that dementia risk is lowest in people who adopt a healthy lifestyle in mid-life by regularly exercising, not smoking, drinking alcohol only in moderation (if at all), and maintaining a healthy weight and diet.

Smoking

Smoking has an extremely harmful effect on the lungs, heart, and vascular system, including the brain's blood vessels. It increases the risk of developing dementia later in life, especially Alzheimer's disease (stroke, type 2 diabetes, and heart disease).

Excessive Consumption of Alcohol

Regularly drinking at high levels over a long period increases a person's risk of developing Alzheimer's disease, vascular Dementia, Korsakoff's syndrome, and alcoholic Dementia.

Improper Diet

An unhealthy or improper diet contains a lot of saturated fat, which raises cholesterol, narrows the arteries, and leads to weight gain. It also includes too much salt (which contributes to high blood pressure and stroke) and too much sugar (an additional factor in weight gain and type 2 diabetes). Along with developing Dementia, an unhealthy diet can affect a person's risk of developing many illnesses, including cardiovascular disease and type 2 diabetes.

Physical Inactivity

This is one of the most vital lifestyle risk factors for developing Dementia, as it directly affects the brain's structure and function.

Acquired Risk Factors

Mid-life hypertension (Mainly responsible for Vascular Dementia)

Disturbed Lipov protein metabolism

Brain Trauma/Head Injuries

CVA/Stroke/TIA

Second-Hand smoking

Physical inactivity

Air pollution (Magnetite Particles/Pesticides/Metals)

Obesity

Hearing impairment

Low education /Occupational Status

Hormonal imbalance (Putting 65% of women at higher risk)

Infections (Pneumonia, Oral Herpes)

People on medications, e.g.

Benzodiazepines

Anticholinergics (Tricyclic antidepressants)

First generation antihistamines.

Bladder Muscarinic (to treat incontinence)

Proton pump inhibitors (Antacids): Omeprazole, Lansoprazole

Other Possible Reasons

Accumulation of Beta Amyloidal plaques

Tau (abnormal build-up of a protein) deposits/tangle throughout the brain

Physical causes (9-19%) include treatable causes like iron deficiency anaemia, pernicious anaemia, thyroid problems, brain tumors', and depression.

(E) Assessments for Dementia

During my career as an occupational therapist, I have noticed that people respond well to questionnaires. This allows a health professional to interpret the dementia stage and results accurately.

Who Should Be Assessed?

All healthcare professionals know there is a high possibility of cognitive impairment in the elderly. However, I have noticed that people take forgetfulness and memory issues very lightly. Caretakers, family, or friends must identify the symptoms we discussed earlier, as they spend the maximum amount of time with the patient. So only if they can identify Dementia will be able to start the treatment.

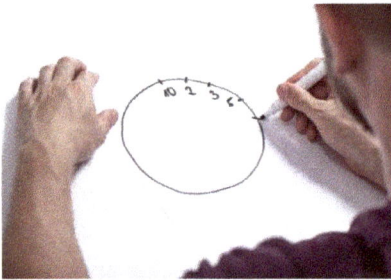

Apart from anyone suffering from the early signs of Dementia or those at higher risk, the following patients should also receive immediate and further evaluation:

- A patient who makes the healthcare professional suspicious of cognitive impairment during the interview.
- A patient who complains of a worsening memory or other cognitive symptoms (unless restricted to naming people).
- A patient where the family or healthcare professional notices difficulties in any of the:
- remembering appointments
- remembering things which recently happened
- recalling conversations
- finding the right words
- taking medication accurately
- dealing with finances
- a decline in personal grooming

- changes in personality
- social withdrawal, loss of interest, or changes in mood
- A patient over 65 years may have been responsible for a car accident.
- An elderly patient who needs to make an essential financial decision (such as selling a house, nominating others to manage financial affairs, or making a will) and mental competence is questioned.

Why Do You Need to Be Assessed?

Getting an assessment done as early as possible can give you several benefits.
For example:

Ruling out the possibility of other medical conditions with similar symptoms, such as urinary tract and chest infections, thyroid problems, severe constipation, vitamin deficiencies, and depression.

Ruling out other possible causes of confusion, such as emotional changes (for example, bereavement or moving house), poor hearing or sight, or the side effects of specific drugs (or drug combinations) you may be taking for other conditions.

Getting an answer to why you are experiencing the symptoms so you can work on managing them.

Get access to any treatments, relevant information, advice, and support (practical, emotional, financial, and legal) you may need.

Moreover, the main benefit of an assessment is that if you are diagnosed with dementia, you will also usually be told what type of dementia and stage it is. However, this cannot always be confirmed.

Do you remember the types of dementia discussed in Chapter A?

Dementia Investigations

Routine Investigations	Reason(s) for the Investigation
Full blood count	To exclude anaemia, infections.
Urea, creatinine and electrolytes	To exclude kidney and metabolic disorders.
Calcium	To exclude high calcium, e.g., due to tumors'.
Liver function tests	To exclude liver failure, liver tumors.
Serum vitamin B12 and red blood cell folate	To exclude deficiency states, pernicious anaemia
Erythrocyte sedimentation rate (ESR)	Often abnormal in inflammatory conditions such as vasculitis and infections.
Thyroid function tests	To exclude overactive and underactive thyroid.
Brain CT scan	To exclude strokes, tumors', subdural hematomas, and hydrocephalus and to determine whether atrophy is present
Chest X-ray	To exclude tumors and infections.

Investigations Required Reason(S) When Clinically Indicated	Reason(s) for the Investigation
Neuropsychological examination	To distinguish mild cognitive impairment from early dementia and to assist in diagnosing the type of dementia.
Brain MRI scan	To exclude vasculitis or encephalopathy and to obtain higher-resolution brain images.
Electrocardiogram (ECG) and Holter monitor	To exclude cardiac causes of vascular dementia
Carotid dopplers	To exclude carotid artery disease as a cause of vascular dementia.
Echocardiogram	To exclude cardiac causes of vascular dementia.
Fasting blood sugar level	To exclude diabetes mellitus
Syphilis serology	To exclude syphilis infection.
Micro urine	To exclude urinary tract infections and renal disease.
Electroencephalogram (EEG)	To exclude epilepsy and encephalopathy
Lumbar puncture	To exclude meningitis or encephalitis.

SPECT or PET scan	To assist in the diagnosis of early Alzheimer's disease and vascular dementia.
Human immunodeficiency virus (HIV) screen	To exclude HIV/AIDS-related disorder
Immunological screen	To exclude vasculitis due to auto-immune disorders.
Genetic screening	For those at risk of Huntington's disease, familial forms of Alzheimer's disease or frontotemporal dementia

Components of Multidisciplinary Dementia Assessment

Medical Assessment

This assessment includes the following examinations:

Mental State Examination: This discovers psychological and cognitive functioning to identify the extent of cognitive deficits and a psychiatric disorder. This mainly includes depression, for which a depression scale is used.

Complete Physical Examination: It focuses mainly on the neurological system.

Complete Medical History: It is usually taken from the patient and the primary informant to understand the problems accurately.

Neuropsychological Assessment

This two to three-hour assessment is performed by a trained neuropsychologist usually available in major centres. They use a battery of standardization evaluate cognitive functions in various areas of the brain. Test scores are compared with population norms; some tests are designed to estimate the procedure before the disease's onset. They are mainly helpful in identifying the pattern of cognitive deficits and in quantifying memory impairment. This may help in determining the type of dementia. If the deficiencies are ambiguous or mild, the test should be repeated in six to twelve months to assess changes not detected by other assessments.

Social Work Assessment

This assessment involves two primary strands. One focuses on the social function and support network of the person with dementia and attempts to determine whether additional social supports are required. The other focuses on the person's family and other caretakers by evaluating their stress level and how well they are coping. In some centres, the latter assessment may be linked with caretaker support groups. The social worker will often be responsible for arranging whatever community services are necessary.

Occupational Therapy Assessment

An advantage of this assessment is that it is usually carried out in the patient's home. It aims to determine their functional capacity by evaluating their ability to perform various day-to-day activities. The assessment concentrates on higher-order activities such as organisational skills, financial management, telephone use, and meal preparation in people with mild cognitive impairments. However, driving evaluations are often undertaken as a separate task.

The assessment covers more basic skills such as toileting, bathing, and dressing in severe deficits. Home basic safety may also be done. For example, if the person has a history of falls, the family and caretakers might be given recommendations about installing rails.

Nursing Assessment

Community nurses perform a combination of cognitive screening and occupational and social work therapy-style assessments in various centres. This is primarily done if the nurse looks after aged patients and those living alone. For them, medication management is a common issue that requires assessment.

Types of Assessments

Some assessments can help you, and your loved ones diagnose dementia. According to my experience, you should get these questionnaires filled out by the older adults in your family. They might be at the early stages, and you surely don't wait for it until the condition deteriorates.

Memory Questionnaire (Mild Dementia)

Read each statement below and mark the box that best describes your current behaviour. It would help to ask someone who knows you well to complete the questionnaire and fill in the independent scorer column.

Scoring: Agree = **2** Partially agree = **1**   Disagree = **0**

Question	Score					
	Self-score			Independent scorer		
	Agree	Partially agree	Disagree	Agree	Partially agree	Disagree
I often need to remember where I have put things in the house.						
I sometimes need help finding a television story or the plot of a						

book.					
I often forget words or find them on the tip of my tongue and cannot quite find them.					
I often forget things and must go back for them.					
I sometimes forget things that I did the day before.					
I forget to do things that I have planned to do.					
I can tell somebody a story or joke that I have said before or ask the same question twice.					

I sometimes forget to tell people important messages.					
I find it challenging to learn a new skill (e.g., working on a computer, a game, or a new gadget) remembering a sequence of instructions.					
I sometimes need help recognising places or people's faces that I have seen before and should be familiar with.					
TOTAL SCORE					

INTERPRETATION

Self-score 8-20: This suggests that you may have a poor memory and benefit from compensatory strategies.

The discrepancy between self-score and independent score

5-20: This indicates that you may not be fully aware of your memory problem or deny it.

AD8 (Dementia Screening Interview) Questionnaire

Remember, "Yes, a change" indicates that there have been changes in the last several years caused by cognitive (memory and thinking) problems.	YES, A change	NO, No change	N/A, Don't know!
1) Problems with judgment (e.g., problems making decisions, bad financial decisions, problems with thinking)			
2) Less interest in hobbies/activities			
3) Repeats the same things over and over (questions, stories, or			

statements)			
4) Trouble learning how to use a tool, appliance, or gadget (e.g., VCR, computer, microwave, remote control)			
5) Forgets the correct month or year			
6) Having trouble handling complicated financial affairs (e.g., balancing a cheque book, income taxes, paying bills)			
7) Trouble remembering appointments			
8) Daily problems with thinking and memory			
TOTAL AD8 SCORE			

INTERPRETATION

The final score is a sum of the items marked "Yes, A change."

Only a screening test is insufficient to diagnose a disorder. However, AD8 is quite sensitive to detecting early cognitive changes associated with many common dementing illnesses. This includes Alzheimer's disease, Lewy body Dementia, Frontotemporal Dementia, and Vascular Dementia.

Scores in the impaired range (see below) indicate a need for further assessment. Scores in the "normal" range suggest a dementing disorder is unlikely, but a very early disease process cannot be ruled out. More advanced assessment may be warranted in cases where other objective evidence of impairment exists.

Based on clinical research findings from 995 individuals included in the development and validation samples, the following cut points are provided:

•   0 – 1: Normal cognition

•   two or greater: Cognitive impairment is likely to be present

What About the Diagnosis?

Why is Diagnosis Important?

A proper medical diagnosis is required if anyone develops dementia-like symptoms and does not appear to get any better.

Diagnosis is important because:

It can rule out the possibility that the symptoms have a different, treatable cause.

If a diagnosis is made, it allows friends, family members, and the person with dementia to make plans.

There are treatments available that may help with some of the symptoms. The sooner you start these treatments, the better.

However, you cannot have dementia and still do everything you used to do. So, part of the diagnosis for dementia is to get a history and to look.

What is this person like now?

Cognitively what are they like?

What are they not able to do now that they used to be able to do before?

Therefore, a person who can still do all those things might have something else, but not dementia. However, there are things that the person cannot do that they used to be able to do. That's what dementia is all about.

Who is Involved in the Diagnosis & Treatment?

If you are worried that you or your loved one might be developing dementia, have your concerns immediately investigated. For this purpose, you will need to meet various healthcare professionals. Each is responsible for a different aspect of care and condition-often termed the multi-professional team approach to dementia.

However, to get the best care possible, it is essential to understand each person's different roles. So, let's dive into it!

General Practitioner (GP)

The first step after suspecting dementia is visiting a General Practitioner. They will ask general questions and assess the concerns on a psychological, social, and physical basis. Even though the GP can diagnose, they usually refer the individual to a specialist for further assessment.

While going to the specialist, a letter will be provided outlining the person's history, social and medical background, and physical examination findings. This may include critical non-medical information such as the number of dependents, occupation, and carer support. In addition, it will give the specialist an idea of the various types of care and support they may require with dementia.

If a diagnosis is made, the specialist will advise the GP, who will take over the ongoing management of the person's care in the community. In the advent of a problem or difficulty, the GP will decide whether they can deal with it- if not, they will refer the person back to the specialist.

Specialists

Geriatrician

A geriatrician is a medical doctor who specialises in diagnosing, treating, and managing diseases of people over 65 years. In addition, they are specialists in treating the deterioration of mental functions and investigating these changes' causes. They work as part of a community-based team that includes social workers, occupational therapists, nurses, and sometimes physiotherapists.

Neurologist

A neurologist is a medical doctor specialising in diagnosing, treating, and managing disorders of the nervous system and brain, especially those that affect consciousness and movement. This includes people who are under 65 years. In addition, they treat and manage conditions relating to the central nervous system, such as epilepsy, Parkinson's disease, migraine, multiple sclerosis, etc. Therefore, they usually work in larger hospitals where the scanning equipment needed for testing is readily available.

Psychiatrist of Old Age (of Later Life)

A psychiatrist of old age is a doctor who specializes in the mental health problems of the elderly. Since dementia is linked to old age, and psychiatrists have significant experience in treating the elderly, they can quickly diagnose dementia and advise on the disease's problems.

Psychiatrist

A psychiatrist is a doctor who specializes in diagnosing and treating various health problems of people under 65 years. Their assessment of a person can be instrumental in cases where severe depression may be causing symptoms similar to those of dementia, making diagnosis difficult.

Clinical Psychologist

A clinical psychologist specializes in assessing learning ability, memory, and other mental functions. For this, they usually conduct an interview, which includes some tests. This allows them better to understand the person's cognitive abilities and difficulties. For treatment, a clinical psychologist often offers counselling and support.

Occupational Therapist

An occupational therapist aims to empower and enable people to stay independent in their daily activities and maintain their physical skills and abilities. This will include determining and analysing ways to compensate or improve for any deficits relating to the symptoms of dementia, such as using the stairs, difficulty getting in or out of a bath, furniture layout, etc. They also give practical advice such as alterations and adaptations to the specialised equipment or home so that people with dementia can become more independent in their daily chores.

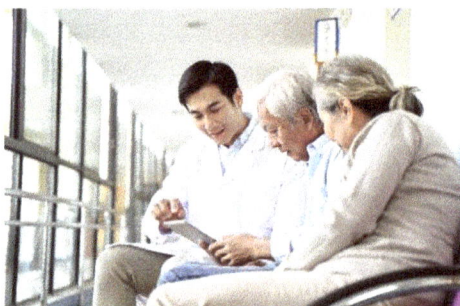

Public Health Nurse

A public health nurse is a qualified general nurse based in the community working out of the local health centre. They do various tasks, such as calling people in their own homes (regularly if required), assessing their needs, and providing support services. In addition, they usually coordinate with a GP and professional nursing duties, such as changing dressings.

Based on an individual's needs, the public health nurse can link to local support by referring to home care and daycare facilities where available. They can also access sub-support such as care attendants, twilight care staff, home help, personal assistants, respite care, and meals on wheels.

Social Worker- Social workers are part of the multi-professional team in the hospital, accessing various statutory and voluntary sectors. Hospital consultants usually refer them to people with dementia and their families.

Social workers' primary role is to determine the needs of the person with dementia and provide skilled psychosocial support to them and their carers while ensuring that the individual is viewed in the context of their overall community environment and family.

What If a Diagnosis Is Made?

 A diagnosis of dementia comes as a shock, no matter how much it is expected. It is hard for the person with the diagnosis and their family to accept, so reassurance and support are imperative. The most important thing is to stay positive and concentrate as much as possible on what you (or the person with dementia) can do rather than what you cannot. Although the person will gradually need more help, it is crucial to ensure that other people don't take over. That independence is preserved as much as possible.

Take time for each other and discuss important matters because now is the time to think about health, legal, financial, and personal affairs and plans for the future. The person may need to make or change the Will, and an Enduring Power of Attorney should be discussed with a solicitor if not already done.

While you are reading this, be assured that you are not alone. You do not have to face dementia by yourself. You can find support from all kinds of people – friends, family, professionals, and volunteers working with people with dementia and others with dementia.

(F) What Can Be Done for Prevention?

While we know that there is no cure for Dementia, for now, we CAN delay the later stages. It can be frightening to think about this disease, especially if you have witnessed a loved one suffering from it. However, even though you may have been told that all you can do is hope for the best and wait for a pharmaceutical cure, the truth is much more encouraging.

Promising research shows that you can reduce your risk of dementia through a combination of simple but effective lifestyle changes. According to experts, the risk is not limited to old age, but it can start in the brain long before symptoms are detected, often in middle age.

That means it's never too early to start taking care of your brain health. The more you start taking precautions from an early age, the longer and stronger your brain will stay working, and the more likely you will be able to reduce your risk of developing Dementia. This includes not smoking/ consuming excessive alcohol, and have a proper diet for blood pressure, sugar, etc.

So why not help yourself and make small changes for a better future? Factors that are modifiable and can contribute to the prevention of Dementia are:

1. Blood Pressure
Most people who take anti-hypertensive medication take it for an extended period without reviewing or consulting with their doctors. It has been revealed that some of those medications can be a contributing factor to iatrogenic Dementia. Therefore, it is recommended that you talk to your doctor and see if they are satisfied with your prescription or want to review them.
2.Diet
A person's diet is essential in deciding the long-term medical conditions they can develop. For Dementia, it is recommended to have a Mediterranean-type diet. It includes the following:

A large proportion of fruits and vegetables(such as legumes, cereals, and beans etc.)

Fish (rich in Omega3), e.g., mackerel, tuna, herring, and salmon.

Dairy products

Nuts

Poultry

Red meat, sugar, and saturated fats are in a minimal amount. Other essential elements that have been reported in preventing Dementia are:

Vitamins and Minerals, e.g., Folic Acid, Vitamin B, 6 & B12, Vitamin D, Magnesium, Vitamin C & E, Oils, e.g., coconut oil, rapeseed oil, olive oil, polyunsaturated & fish related fats.

3. Diabetes
Since uncontrolled diabetes is also a significant contributor to Dementia, it would be advisable to check your sugar levels even if you are on the borderline.
4. Alcohol
Excessive alcohol consumption is also a contributing factor in Dementia. Therefore, if you consume alcohol, make sure that you take it in moderation.
5. Habits
A person's habits significantly contribute to preventing or causing a long-term condition like Dementia, diabetes, stress, anxiety, or depression. Concerning Dementia, it recommended that you do the following:
Keep a routine for your activities.

Keep yourself active through your interest activities, as physical activity counteracts the presence of a significant contributing factor (Apo E4) in the blood.

Meet people, socialise and stay positive. Did you know laughing is reported to be associated with boosting your immunity?

Talk to people if you are finding some difficulty in your life. It can either be a family member, friend, or professional. Of course, it's always better to let things out instead of overthinking.

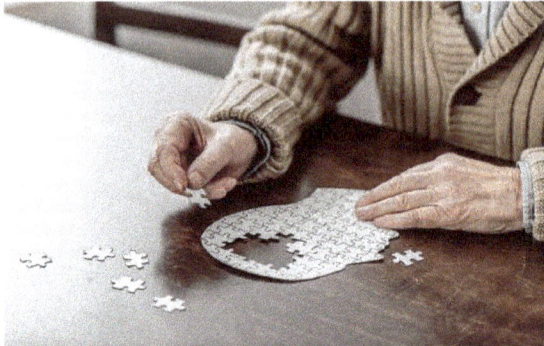

Keep a record of your good memories. Then, whenever you feel sad or stressed out, going through old memories will undoubtedly bring a smile to your face!

Keep a scheduled time to sleep and relax. Always remember to take breaks and not overwork. It will make you over exerted. Your brain will keep working while you sleep. This will affect your brain activity in the long term, which could welcome Dementia.

Watch the food you are eating and keep yourself hydrated.

Make a habit of reading, e.g., newspapers, magazines, and books.

Write down things that are important to you. Then, keep a diary and write anything you in it at the end of the day – something to do for the next day, reminders, etc.

Plans for the future and change roles (Assistive decision making).

Learning a new language or watching a movie in a different language.

6. Hormonal Imbalance

It is also reported to be a risk factor in rising cases of Dementia, especially in females. Therefore, it would be advisable not to ignore symptoms and consult your doctor if needed.

7. Sleep

Sleep is one of the major contributors to causing Dementia. Since it helps recharge your body and mind, it would be great to be mindful of your sleep timing and duration. However, lack of sleep should not be ignored; if you face difficulties in sleeping, you should discuss it with your doctor.
Find some useful strategies below:

- Always sleep around the same time.
- Keep bedroom temperature lower than your living room.
- Go to bed without any distractions like phones or books.
- Do not drink coffee or tea before bed, as they contain caffeine, which can disturb your sleeping pattern.
- Keep a bottle of water near the bed to drink at night.
- Try to keep the bedroom completely dark or use a dim light bulb.

8. Smoking

Never start smoking because it's challenging to quit the habit. If possible, avoid sitting in the company of people who smoke, as second-hand smoke & air pollution are listed as one of contributing risk factors in Dementia.

9. Socialization

As per research, socially active & engaged people are less likely to develop symptoms of Dementia.

10. Stress Management

Long-term stress without intervention has the potential to contribute to developing Dementia. Some of the most used strategies in stress management:

Yoga

Meditation

Mindfulness

Walk

Exercise

Gym

11. Physical Fitness

Aerobic exercise or any other, at least three times a week, is reported to help prevent Dementia.

12. Lifelong Learning

According to studies, people who keep their brains active are the least vulnerable group concerning Dementia. Hence, you can choose what keeps your brain busy like:

- Learn a new language.
- Learn music.
- Read newspapers or Magazines.
- Solve puzzles or play Sudoku.
- Play cards and talk to your friends or family.
- Watch news or TV programs and then discuss them with others.
- Write a paragraph every day if you can.
- Write a journal daily, and summarise the day, if you can. Develop a habit of writing your tasks for the day.

(G) How to Manage Dementia Clients?

Ways to Help the Memory

If you face difficulty remembering things and are in the earlier stages of dementia, help yourself before it gets too late. Since different things help different people, you can choose the ones that suit you.

Here are some things you can do:

Make a Timetable

Structure your day by making a timetable and setting a routine. It will remind you what you need to do during the day, make you feel productive, and, most importantly, keep your brain functioning.

Keep Things in The Same Place

Put things of regular use in the same place where they are easy

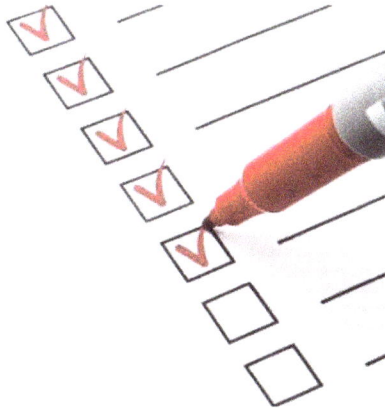

to see. This will help you keep track of things like your wallet, keys, phone, glasses, medicines, etc.

Write It Down

Many people find a wall calendar and wipe-clean board in their kitchen helpful. You and your family can write down important things about a particular day and check what remains for the day.

Make A Checklist of Essential Things to Do Before Going Out and Before Going to Bed.

Leave the checklist at the front door or on your nightstand. Always check that you have done everything on your list each time you leave the house.

Make To-Do Notes or Lists.

Make lists using to-do lists, planners, or sticky notes to remember what you must do during the day. You can also put notes near an appliance, remote control, front door, or bedside table.

Track Your Daily Routine with a Calendar or Diary

Keep the calendar or diary in a place that is easy to see or check each day- so that it becomes part of your daily routine.

You can also use The Daily Schedule tracker below for this purpose.

Monday	
Tuesday	
Wednesday	
Thursday	
Friday	
Saturday	
Sunday	

Keep Phone Numbers Where They Are Easy to Find

Keep important phone numbers, a notepad, and a pen near your mobile so you can find them easily and quickly whenever you need them. You can also use photos or mobile phones to make it easier to call certain people.

You might include:

Emergency numbers for gas, water, electricity

GP, local hospital, community services

local stations

local plumber, builder, electrician, minicab, or taxi service

numbers of your close relatives and friends

Telephone Prompt Card

- · **Write all messages down.**
- · **Tell the caller that you are writing the message down.**
- · **Read the message back to the caller.**

Date: **Time:**

Caller: **Caller's Number**

Message:

Whenever you talk to someone on call, you can use a telephone message prompt sheet like the one below to ensure you get all the important messages.

Organise Your Medication

Keep your medications in a pillbox or medication organiser. It will enable you to keep track of your different medicines, and you won't skip medicine any day. You can also use a Medication Management Chart like the one below.

Medication Management Chart

	Name of Meds	Mon	Tues	Wed	Thurs	Fri	Sat	Sun
Morning								
Lunchtime								
Dinner time								
Night-time								

Use Technology and Equipment

Technology and equipment can help you to live more independently. They can also help provide reassurance and support and reduce the risk of accidents. For example, they can help you to:

remember dates, days, and time.

take medication on time.

identify if gas is left on.

let people know where you are if you get lost.

How to Ensure Safety?

If you have been diagnosed with dementia or know a loved one suffering from it, here's a safety checklist that will allow them to do everything to ensure their safety. You can keep it on your mobile, front door, or nightstand for easy access.

The Safety Checklist

Dining Room	Check Front Doors are closed and locked.
	Always ask before opening the door.
	Do not open to strangers.
	Check fire is switched off.
	Check TV is switched off.
Kitchen	Check Back door is locked.
	Check that windows are closed.
	Check cooker is turned off.
	Check taps are turned off.
Lounge	Check that windows are closed and locked.
	Check front windows are closed.
Downstairs bathroom	Check that windows are closed.
	Check taps are turned off.
Hall	Check front door is locked.
Bedroom	Ensure the electric blanket is turned off

If going away	Unplug appliances
	Turn off heating
	Make sure doors and windows are locked.

In addition to the essential precautions and checklist that you just read, when caring for someone with dementia, you require the right balance between protecting them for the sake of safety and encouraging independence. Rather than curtailing their freedom, you may need to accept that minor accidents may occur. But there are some more sensible precautions you can take.

Lighting

> ➢ Make sure the lighting is bright.
> ➢ The hall should be well-lighted.
> ➢ If the person with dementia is likely to get up during the night, use a night light in the bedroom.

Aids

Aids such as handrails in the stairs, hall, toilet, or bath will assist the person if they are unsteady on their feet.

Falls

Falls are common among older people and can be dangerous. Check the home for anything that may result in a fall, such as:

> ➢ broken stair rods
> ➢ lose carpet, especially on the stairs.
> ➢ loose mats
> ➢ slippery or highly-polished floors
> ➢ trailing flexes

➤ unsteady furniture
➤ old, lost, or worn footwear
➤ clutter or objects that are lying on the floor.

If you or the dementia patient in your house has a serious fall, do not try to move them or give them anything to drink if they need anesthesia. Instead, keep them warm and call an ambulance immediately.

Dangerous Substances

➤ After taking medicine, put them somewhere safe if they forget and take an extra dose.
➤ Lock all poisonous substances, such as disinfectant, paint strippers, and cleaning fluids, in case someone with dementia accidentally drinks them.
➤ Call an ambulance or take them immediately to the nearest accident and emergency department if you think someone may have swallowed something poisonous. Take the container and the remains of any substance with you to help the doctor decide what treatment to give.

Kitchen

➤ Place items in everyday use in easy reach, so they do not have to climb on a chair or stretch to get them.
➤ Keep away sharp knives or appliances that the person can no longer safely use.
➤ Use an electric kettle that switches itself off once it has boiled.
➤ Fit an isolation valve with a 'nursery' switch to a gas cooker to prevent them from turning on the oven when you are out.
➤ If the person burns or scalds themselves, pour cold water over the affected area for at least ten minutes to reduce the skin's heat and pain. Remove anything tight, such as rings or watches, as burnt skin can swell. Do not apply ointment. Cover with a clean non-fluffy cloth and contact

the GP or take the person to the nearest emergency and accident department.

Heating

➢ Since heaters or fires can be dangerous for someone with dementia, they should always have a fixed guard.
➢ Never dry clothes over a heater or fire, as this can cause a fire.
➢ Never bring a portable electric heater into the bathroom, as it could be fatal.
➢ If you are using a gas water heater, ensure it is serviced regularly and that the room is well-ventilated.
➢ You can fit an isolation valve and 'nursery' switch to a gas fire to prevent someone from turning it on while you are out.
➢ You can regulate central heating and many electric fires with a time switch.
➢ Cold is a genuine risk. Many older people become chilled without noticing. If it is necessary to economize on heating, it may be better for the person to live in one room which can be well heated during cold spells.
➢ Put the bed against an inner wall, as that will be warmer.
➢ Use draught-proof doors and windows.
➢ Put sheets of newspaper under the floor covering to give added protection from cold.
➢ A quarter of a building's heat is lost through the roof, so a grant may be available if your house has an attic that has yet to be insulated (Especially in Europe).

Other Precautions

➢ If gas is used,
➢ Fitting gas detectors and smoke alarms are helpful if other people are in the home. However, a person with dementia may not know what the alarm sound means.
➢ A person with dementia should avoid using an electric blanket if there is any risk of incontinence.

> ➤ If the person with dementia smokes, ensure they do not drop cigarettes or lit matches.

Seek Help from Neighbors

Lastly, if you or the patient live on your own and the carer or family members are out for a prolonged period, a friendly neighbour may be able to watch out for signs that something may be wrong. Leave a phone number and a set of spare keys with them where you can be contacted.

Are You a Carer?

If you are a carer and have no clue about the client's personality and needs, and the client cannot communicate at the later stages of dementia, they can get agitated.

Therefore, it would be best to first discuss with the patient's family to know the patient. You can also make a questionnaire like the one below and fill it out.

Questions	Answers
1. How much salt do they prefer in their food?	
2. Do they prefer hot or warm tea, and with how much sugar?	
3. What do they enjoy the most?	
4. What makes them angry?	
5. How much temperature of the room is okay for them?	
6. What type of clothes do they prefer?	
7. What is their food habit and timings?	

8. Do they like the company of people?	
9. Do they prefer company or solitary?	

The Grocery List Template

As we have already discussed, taking care of dementia patients shouldn't remove all their independence. With a bit of help, dementia patients can carry out their daily tasks in hassle-free; check out the grocery lists ahead!

Grocery List Template

Grocery List

Fruit and Veg

- ☐ _____ ☐ _____
- ☐ _____ ☐ _____
- ☐ _____ ☐ _____
- ☐ _____ ☐ _____

Bread & Baking [bread, buns, flour, mixes, yeast, powder]

- ☐ _____ ☐ _____
- ☐ _____ ☐ _____
- ☐ _____ ☐ _____
- ☐ _____ ☐ _____

Fridge Section [meat, milk, eggs, cheese, cream]

- ☐ _____ ☐ _____
- ☐ _____ ☐ _____
- ☐ _____ ☐ _____
- ☐ _____ ☐ _____

Snacks & Drinks [juice, tea, coffee, crackers, sweets]

- ☐ _____ ☐ _____
- ☐ _____ ☐ _____
- ☐ _____ ☐ _____

Tinned Foods [soup, tuna, beans, fruits, vegetables]

- ☐ _____ ☐ _____
- ☐ _____ ☐ _____
- ☐ _____ ☐ _____

Dry Foods [cereal, pasta, rice, sugar, oatmeal, mixes]

- ☐ _____ ☐ _____
- ☐ _____ ☐ _____
- ☐ _____ ☐ _____
- ☐ _____ ☐ _____

Frozen [ice, vegetables, chicken, desserts, juice, pizza]

- ☐ _____ ☐ _____
- ☐ _____ ☐ _____
- ☐ _____ ☐ _____
- ☐ _____ ☐ _____

Condiments & Spices [ketchup, jam, mayo, dressing]

- ☐ _____ ☐ _____
- ☐ _____ ☐ _____

Pet

- ☐ _____ ☐ _____

Supplies [paper & plastic, cleaning, personal, health]

- ☐ _____ ☐ _____
- ☐ _____ ☐ _____
- ☐ _____ ☐ _____
- ☐ _____ ☐ _____
- ☐ _____ ☐ _____
- ☐ _____ ☐ _____

Miscellaneous & Other

- ☐ _____ ☐ _____
- ☐ _____ ☐ _____
- ☐ _____ ☐ _____
- ☐ _____ ☐ _____

Grocery List

Fruit and Veg

- ☐ _____ ☐ _____
- ☐ _____ ☐ _____
- ☐ _____ ☐ _____
- ☐ _____ ☐ _____

Bread & Baking [bread, buns, flour, mixes, yeast, powder]

- ☐ _____ ☐ _____
- ☐ _____ ☐ _____
- ☐ _____ ☐ _____
- ☐ _____ ☐ _____

Fridge Section [meat, milk, eggs, cheese, cream]

- ☐ _____ ☐ _____
- ☐ _____ ☐ _____
- ☐ _____ ☐ _____
- ☐ _____ ☐ _____

Snacks & Drinks [juice, tea, coffee, crackers, sweets]

- ☐ _____ ☐ _____
- ☐ _____ ☐ _____
- ☐ _____ ☐ _____

Tinned Foods [soup, tuna, beans, fruits, vegetables]

- ☐ _____ ☐ _____
- ☐ _____ ☐ _____
- ☐ _____ ☐ _____

Dry Foods [cereal, pasta, rice, sugar, oatmeal, mixes]

- ☐ _____ ☐ _____
- ☐ _____ ☐ _____
- ☐ _____ ☐ _____
- ☐ _____ ☐ _____

Frozen [ice, vegetables, chicken, desserts, juice, pizza]

- ☐ _____ ☐ _____
- ☐ _____ ☐ _____
- ☐ _____ ☐ _____
- ☐ _____ ☐ _____

Condiments & Spices [ketchup, jam, mayo, dressing]

- ☐ _____ ☐ _____
- ☐ _____ ☐ _____

Pet

- ☐ _____ ☐ _____

Supplies [paper & plastic, cleaning, personal, health]

- ☐ _____ ☐ _____
- ☐ _____ ☐ _____
- ☐ _____ ☐ _____
- ☐ _____ ☐ _____
- ☐ _____ ☐ _____
- ☐ _____ ☐ _____

Miscellaneous & Other

- ☐ _____ ☐ _____
- ☐ _____ ☐ _____
- ☐ _____ ☐ _____
- ☐ _____ ☐ _____

CRITICAL
- ☐
- ☐
- ☐
- ☐
- ☐

PRODUCE
- ☐ Apples
- ☐ Avocados
- ☐ Bananas
- ☐ Berries
- ☐ Broccoli
- ☐ Carrots
- ☐ Celery
- ☐ Cucumbers
- ☐ Garlic
- ☐ Grapefruit
- ☐ Grapes
- ☐ Lemons/Limes
- ☐ Lettuce
- ☐ Melons
- ☐ Mushrooms
- ☐ Onions
- ☐ Oranges
- ☐ Peppers
- ☐ Potatoes
- ☐ Squash/Zucchini
- ☐ Tomatoes
- ☐
- ☐

BREAD / BAKERY
- ☐ Bagels
- ☐ Bread
- ☐ Cake
- ☐ Cookies
- ☐ Dinner Rolls
- ☐ Donuts
- ☐ French Bread
- ☐ Hamburger Buns
- ☐ Hot Dog Buns
- ☐ Muffins
- ☐ Pastries
- ☐ Pie
- ☐ Pita Bread
- ☐ Tortillas
- ☐
- ☐

BREAKFAST
- ☐ Cold Cereal
- ☐ Oatmeal
- ☐ Creamed Wheat
- ☐ Pancake Mix
- ☐
- ☐

MEAT
- ☐ Bacon
- ☐ Beef / Steak
- ☐ Chicken
- ☐ Deli Meat
- ☐ Fish
- ☐ Ground Beef
- ☐ Ham
- ☐ Hot Dogs
- ☐ Pork
- ☐ Sausage
- ☐ Turkey
- ☐
- ☐

DAIRY / FRIDGE
- ☐ Biscuits
- ☐ Butter
- ☐ Cheese
- ☐ Cookie Dough
- ☐ Cream Cheese
- ☐ Dips
- ☐ Eggs
- ☐ Half & Half
- ☐ Milk
- ☐ Sour Cream
- ☐ Whip Cream
- ☐ Yogurt
- ☐
- ☐

FROZEN
- ☐ Chicken
- ☐ Desserts
- ☐ Dinners
- ☐ Fish
- ☐ Fruits
- ☐ Ice
- ☐ Ice Cream
- ☐ Ice Pops
- ☐ Juice
- ☐ Lasagna
- ☐ Pie
- ☐ Pizza
- ☐ Vegetables
- ☐ Waffles
- ☐

DRINKS
- ☐ Water
- ☐ Juice
- ☐ Soda
- ☐ Sports Drinks
- ☐ Coffee
- ☐ Tea
- ☐
- ☐

CANNED
- ☐ Applesauce
- ☐ Beans
- ☐ Chili
- ☐ Fruits
- ☐ Mushrooms
- ☐ Olives
- ☐ Soup
- ☐ Tomato Sauce
- ☐ Tuna
- ☐ Vegetables
- ☐
- ☐
- ☐
- ☐

DRY / BAKING
- ☐ Baking Powder
- ☐ Baking Soda
- ☐ Bread Crumbs
- ☐ Brownie Mix
- ☐ Cake Mix
- ☐ Canned Milk
- ☐ Chocolate Chips
- ☐ Cocoa
- ☐ Cornmeal
- ☐ Cornstarch
- ☐ Flour
- ☐ Food Coloring
- ☐ Frosting
- ☐ Muffin Mix
- ☐ Oatmeal
- ☐ Pie Crust
- ☐ Shortening
- ☐ Sugar (brown)
- ☐ Sugar (powder)
- ☐ Sugar (white)
- ☐ Vanilla
- ☐ Yeast
- ☐
- ☐

PASTA / RICE
- ☐ Couscous
- ☐ Hamburger Helper
- ☐ Lasagna
- ☐ Mac & Cheese
- ☐ Macaroni
- ☐ Noodle Mixes
- ☐ Ramen
- ☐ Rice (brown)
- ☐ Rice (white)
- ☐ Rice Mixes
- ☐ Spaghetti
- ☐
- ☐
- ☐

SAUCES / OILS
- ☐ Vegetable Oil
- ☐ Soy Sauce
- ☐ Olive Oil
- ☐ Vinegar
- ☐ BBQ Sauce
- ☐ Hot Sauce
- ☐ Spaghetti Sauce
- ☐ Syrup
- ☐

CONDIMENTS
- ☐ Croutons
- ☐ Honey
- ☐ Jam / Jelly
- ☐ Ketchup
- ☐ Mayonnaise
- ☐ Mustard
- ☐ Peanut Butter
- ☐ Pickles
- ☐ Salad Dressing
- ☐ Salsa
- ☐
- ☐

SPICES
- ☐ Salt
- ☐ Pepper
- ☐ Cinnamon
- ☐
- ☐

SNACKS
- ☐ Candy
- ☐ Cookies
- ☐ Crackers
- ☐ Dip / Salsa
- ☐ Dried Fruits
- ☐ Fruit Snacks
- ☐ Graham Crackers
- ☐ Granola Bars
- ☐ Nuts / Seeds
- ☐ Popcorn
- ☐ Potato Chips
- ☐ Pretzels
- ☐ Pudding
- ☐ Raisins
- ☐ Tortilla Chips
- ☐

BABY
- ☐ Baby Food
- ☐ Diapers
- ☐ Formula
- ☐ Rash Cream
- ☐ Wipes
- ☐

PERSONAL
- ☐ Conditioner
- ☐ Cotton Products
- ☐ Deodorant
- ☐ Feminine
- ☐ Floss
- ☐ Hair Spray
- ☐ Lip Balm
- ☐ Lotion
- ☐ Makeup
- ☐ Mouthwash
- ☐ Pain Relievers
- ☐ Razor Blades
- ☐ Shampoo
- ☐ Shaving Cream
- ☐ Soap
- ☐ Sunscreen
- ☐ Toothbrush
- ☐ Toothpaste
- ☐

PAPER / PLASTIC
- ☐ Aluminum Foil
- ☐ Bags
- ☐ Coffee Filters
- ☐ Cups
- ☐ Garbage Bags
- ☐ Napkins
- ☐ Paper Towels
- ☐ Plastic Wrap
- ☐ Plates
- ☐ Tissues
- ☐ Toilet Paper
- ☐ Utensils
- ☐ Wax Paper
- ☐

HOUSEHOLD
- ☐ Batteries
- ☐ Bleach
- ☐ Cards
- ☐ Charcoal
- ☐ Detergent
- ☐ Dish Soap
- ☐ Dishwasher Soap
- ☐ Fabric Softener
- ☐ Glass Cleaner
- ☐ Light Bulbs
- ☐ Rags
- ☐ Sponges
- ☐ Vacuum Bags
- ☐

PET
- ☐ Pet Food
- ☐ Cat Litter
- ☐ Treats

Shopping List Template

Shopping List

- [ ] _____
- [ ] _____
- [ ] _____
- [ ] _____
- [ ] _____
- [ ] _____
- [ ] _____
- [ ] _____
- [ ] _____
- [ ] _____
- [ ] _____
- [ ] _____
- [ ] _____
- [ ] _____
- [ ] _____
- [ ] _____
- [ ] _____
- [ ] _____
- [ ] _____
- [ ] _____
- [ ] _____
- [ ] _____
- [ ] _____
- [ ] _____
- [ ] _____
- [ ] _____
- [ ] _____
- [ ] _____
- [ ] _____
- [ ] _____
- [ ] _____
- [ ] _____
- [ ] _____
- [ ] _____
- [ ] _____
- [ ] _____
- [ ] _____

Shopping List

- [ ] _____
- [ ] _____
- [ ] _____
- [ ] _____
- [ ] _____
- [ ] _____
- [ ] _____
- [ ] _____
- [ ] _____
- [ ] _____
- [ ] _____
- [ ] _____
- [ ] _____
- [ ] _____
- [ ] _____
- [ ] _____
- [ ] _____
- [ ] _____
- [ ] _____
- [ ] _____
- [ ] _____
- [ ] _____
- [ ] _____
- [ ] _____
- [ ] _____
- [ ] _____
- [ ] _____
- [ ] _____
- [ ] _____
- [ ] _____
- [ ] _____
- [ ] _____
- [ ] _____
- [ ] _____
- [ ] _____
- [ ] _____
- [ ] _____

Shopping List

- [ ] _____
- [ ] _____
- [ ] _____
- [ ] _____
- [ ] _____
- [ ] _____
- [ ] _____
- [ ] _____
- [ ] _____
- [ ] _____
- [ ] _____
- [ ] _____
- [ ] _____
- [ ] _____
- [ ] _____
- [ ] _____
- [ ] _____
- [ ] _____
- [ ] _____
- [ ] _____
- [ ] _____
- [ ] _____
- [ ] _____
- [ ] _____
- [ ] _____
- [ ] _____
- [ ] _____
- [ ] _____
- [ ] _____
- [ ] _____
- [ ] _____
- [ ] _____
- [ ] _____
- [ ] _____
- [ ] _____
- [ ] _____

How Can You Monitor the Behavior?

Behaviour Checklist

Client Name: _____

Family Carer: _____

Changes to Emotional Reactions/Attitudes	Change noted?	Source of stress?
Level of Interest: Has s/he lost interest in seeing people or doing things?		
Level of Prompting: Does s/he need prompting to start and continue activities?		
Repetition: Does s/he repeat actions or remarks?		
Attention: Is s/he easily distractible, disorganized, indecisive, or unable to complete a task?		
Flexibility to change: Does s/he appear stubborn or rigid in thinking lately? Are there any obsessive routines or behaviours?		
Judgment/Impulsivity: Has s/he acted impulsively, irresponsibly, or in poor judgment in decisions, spending or driving?		
Insight: Does s/he seem unaware of any problems or changes in behaviour or deny them when discussed?		

	Change noted?	Source of stress?
Type of emotional response: Does s/he respond differently to occasions of joy or sadness		
Irritability: Has s/he been unusually irritable, short-tempered?		

Communication and Social Skill	Change noted?	Source of stress?
Level of Speech: Is s/he less talkative than before?		
Quality of language: Does s/he make language or pronunciation errors, or has s/he developed stuttering or grammatical errors recently?		
Comprehension: Does s/he have trouble comprehending words or objects?		
Social Inappropriateness: Has she/he said or done socially inappropriate things, like being rude/childish? Has s/he been making jokes excessively/ offensively or at the wrong time?		

Comments:

_____

_____

_____

_____

_____

Activity and Behaviour Changes	Change noted?	Source of stress?
Personal Hygiene: Does s/he neglect to wash or change his/her clothes?		
Hoarding: Has s/he started to hoard objects or money excessively?		
Restlessness: Has s/he been roaming, pacing, walking, or driving excessively?		
Aggression: Has s/he shown aggression, shouted at anyone, or hurt anyone physically?		
Clumsiness: Has s/he developed clumsiness, inability to use utensils or appliances, or does a hand interfere with the other?		
Food Habits: Has she/he been drinking or overeating, developing food fads, or putting objects in his/her mouth?		
Inappropriate Sexual behaviours: Has she/he made sexual remarks or undressed in an unusual or excessive situation?		
Fidgeting: Does she/he seem to need to touch, feel, examine, or pick up objects within reach and sight?		

Incontinence: Have they wet or soiled themselves? (Unrelated to other medical diagnoses?)		

Comments:

_____

_____

_____

_____

_____

_____

_____

_____

_____

_____

How Can you Help Someone with Dementia?

Emotionally and Physically

A person with dementia with declining mental abilities will always feel helpless and require encouragement and care. Those around them need to do everything they can to help them retain their sense of identity and their feelings of self-worth.

Carers and family should remember that:

Each person with dementia is a unique individual with their own very different experiences of life, their own needs and feelings, and their likes and dislikes.

Each person will be affected by their dementia differently.

Everyone reacts to the experience of dementia in a different way. This is because experience means other things to different people.

Those caring for people with dementia will need to consider the interests, preferences, and abilities they have at present and the

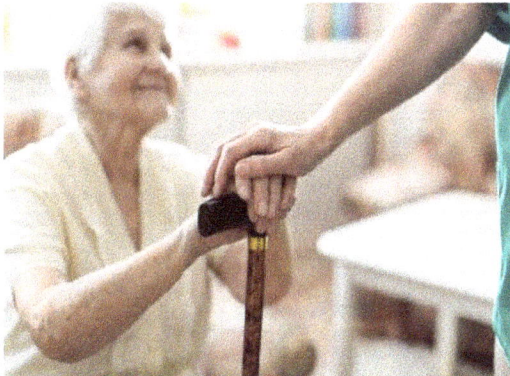

fact that these may change as dementia progresses. Therefore, they should be prepared to respond sensitively, flexibly, and repetitively.

Background Information

If you are hiring a career, give them some background information about their past and present situation. Then, it will be easier for others to see them as a whole rather than merely as someone with dementia. Moreover, carers will be able to connect with them and allow them to trust you. Furthermore, you will feel more confident about finding conversation topics or suggesting activities that the person may enjoy.

It would be best if you reminded others that:

Dementia is nothing to be ashamed of, and it is no one's fault.

Dementia may cause the person to behave in ways others find irritating or upsetting, but this is not deliberate behaviour.

People with dementia often remember the past far more clearly than the recent present and are usually happy to talk about their memories (unless these are painful).

Remember Their Names

Our sense of who we are is closely connected to the name or names we are known by. Therefore, it is ensured that others address the person with dementia in a way they recognise and prefer. Only some people are happy for other people to call them by their first name or the name used by friends and family. Some may choose younger people or those who do not know them well to use a courtesy title such as 'Mr.' or 'Mrs.

Know Their Culture and Religion

Make sure that the carer has appropriate and sufficient details about any relevant cultural or religious customs or beliefs so that these can be respected. It may include anything from clothing, diet, and the use of jewelry to undressing, doing hair, washing, or going to the toilet.

Do not Infantilize Them.

Everyone must continue to treat the person as an adult and with courtesy, irrespective of how advanced their dementia is. Likewise, regardless of how much the person with dementia can or cannot understand, it would be best to be respectful.

Be kind and reassuring without talking down to the person with dementia as though they are a small child.

Never talk over the head of a person with dementia or across them as though they are not there.

Please do not talk about the person with dementia in front of them unless they are included in the conversation.

Avoid scolding or criticising the person, as this will make them feel small.

Look for the meaning behind what they may be trying to communicate, even if it does not make sense.

Be Patient with Them

You must have patience while working with a dementia patient. They can often get easily confused, startled, or agitated. Give them plenty of time to speak, and don't argue with them when they see something that is not there. Try to embrace what they do remember instead of attempting to correct them on what they don't.

Focus on Their Abilities

Help the person avoid situations they are bound to fail since this can be humiliating. Instead, look for tasks they can still manage and activities they can still enjoy.

Praise and encourage them and let them do things at their own pace and in their way.

Do things with the person rather than for them so that they can maintain some independence.

Break activities into small steps to feel achievement, even if they can only manage part of a task.

Much of our self-respect is often bound up in the way we look. Therefore, encourage the person to take pride in their appearance and give them plenty of praise.

Help Them Have a Social Life

People with dementia should continue to enjoy their interests and hobbies as much as possible.
You can offer support by:
> including them in social events and activities
> involving them in an activity, they enjoy
> encouraging them to join a conversation.
> taking them to their favourite place
> let them do their favourite activity, such as gardening.

Please respect Their Privacy.

Try to make sure that the person's right to privacy is respected.

For example, suggest that people knock on their bedroom door before entering.

If the person needs help with intimate activities such as washing or going to the toilet, this should be done sensitively. For example, ensure that the bathroom door is closed if other people are around.

Offer a Choice

The person with dementia must be informed and, wherever possible, consulted about matters which concern them. They should also be given every opportunity to make appropriate choices.

Even if you still determine how much the person can understand, always explain what you are doing and why. You may then be able to judge their reaction from their expression or body language.

Although too many choices can be confusing, you can continue to offer options by phrasing questions that only need a 'yes' or 'no' answer, such as 'Would you like to wear your blue jumper today?'

Allow Them to Express Their Feelings

Dementia affects the thinking and reasoning part of the brain and memory. It does not mean that the person no longer has feelings. People with dementia are likely to be sad or upset at times. They have the right to expect those caring to understand how they feel and make time to offer support rather than ignoring them.

People may want to talk about their anxieties and problems in the earlier stages. Instead of changing the topic, listening and showing that they are there for them is essential.

Respect and Value Them

Dementia patients need to feel respected and valued for who they are now and who they were in the past. It helps if those caring:

are tolerant and flexible.

can make time to chat, listen, enjoy being with the person and show appropriate affection.

Financials

When diagnosing Alzheimer's or related dementia has been made, several important legal and financial issues should be considered as early as possible.

Joint Bank Accounts

Joint bank accounts help deal with the financial affairs of people with mobility problems or those unable to manage a report independently. Any person can open a bank account when that person has the necessary mental capacity (which may be when a person is diagnosed with early-stage dementia).

When an account is opened, an account holder may authorise the bank to accept cheques if another individual sign. However, suppose one account holder becomes mentally incapacitated. In that case, the legal authority to operate the account may be revoked, and it may not be possible for the account to be used by the other joint account holder.

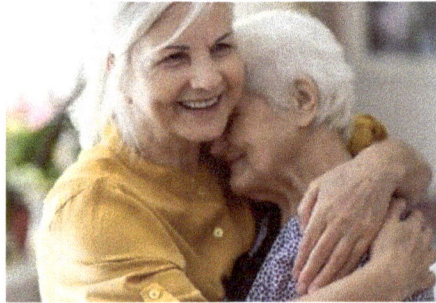

Agency Arrangements for Social Welfare Payments

The Department of Social, Community and Family Affairs has the power to make payments to a third party acting on behalf of the recipient. The person to whom a social welfare benefit is payable may nominate another person to receive that benefit on their behalf. However, the person appointed (agent) has no power to deal with other financial matters.

Make a Will

A Will is a written document in which a person sets out legally binding wishes about the distribution of an estate after death. Dementia patients should be encouraged to make a Will as early as possible, disposing of their estate. However, before this, a doctor should certify that the person with dementia is still mentally capable of understanding and making such a document. If they are married, their spouse should also make a Will.

> ➢ Having a Will is important because it not only delivers the details for the disposal of the money or property but can also:
> ➢ Express burial wishes and any other details concerning funeral arrangements or the disposal of the body.
> ➢ Save next of kin or other beneficiaries substantial inheritance tax.
> ➢ Appoint guardians for any children under eighteen if one or both spouses die in an accident.
> ➢ Leave specific assets to specific children or beneficiaries and specify that certain heirs can only inherit property at 21 or older.
> ➢ Even though anyone can draw up a Will, it is best to go to a solicitor as they are experienced in this work. It will also reduce the probability of Will being challenged after the person's death.

Enduring Power of Attorney (EPA)

An Enduring Power of Attorney (EPA) is a legal arrangement whereby one person (the donor) gives authority to another or others to act on their behalf if the donor becomes mentally incapable of managing their own affairs.

As long as the donor is well, the attorney cannot act upon the EPA. A person can only grant an EPA if they can understand what it is and what it is intended to do. It is still possible for someone to give an EPA after dementia has been diagnosed so long as it is clear that they are fully aware of what is involved.

The GP or consultant will be required to provide a statement that, in their opinion, the donor had the mental capacity at the time of execution to understand the effect of creating an EPA. If this is in question, it may be necessary to have the document signed by the donor in the presence of both the solicitor and the doctor.

Trusts

Trusts are another way of handling another person's financial affairs, whether or not that person is incapable of dealing with their matters. A Trust exists where a person (the trustee) holds the property of another (the settlor) for the benefit of named people (the beneficiaries). The beneficiaries may be the settlor or other people.

Trustees hold and manage the trust property and usually have powers to purchase assets and services for the beneficiaries' use or benefit rather than handing over the money. There is no supervision of the trustees' conduct if they carry out the trust terms.

Covenants

In certain circumstances, an individual may claim relief against an income tax assessment if they make payments through a covenant to another person.

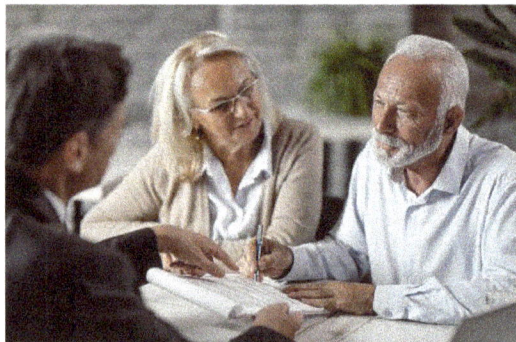

A Deed of Covenant is a legal document under which one person agrees to pay a certain sum each year to another person. The advantage is that the person delivering the money can effectively not pay tax on it. The money is transferred to someone who does not have a taxable income or pays a lower tax rate than the person giving the money. To qualify for relief, there must be a legal obligation to covenant a sum of money for a period that is more than six years.

The circumstances in which an older person can receive sums that are deductible from the covenanter's income are:

if that individual is permanently incapacitated (mentally or physically)

if that individual is over 65 years of age

through payments, which are part of a maintenance agreement between separated spouses.

Tax Relief on Nursing Home Fees for Dependent Relatives

When a family member contributes to maintaining their loved one in a nursing home, it may be possible to claim tax relief on the payments and any other additional medical expenses the person may have. Tax relief for nursing home expenses is claimed under the general scheme for tax relief on certain medical expenses.

 Most nursing homes are approved for tax relief. However, you should contact your local tax office to discuss the specific situation and request the appropriate forms for making a claim.

Activities for People with Dementia

Why Do You Need an Activity?

Getting involved in some purposeful activity is essential for everyone.

Activity is essential to human existence, health, and well-being, meeting inclusion, identity, and life roles.

The urge to engage in purposeful and meaningful activity is a primary human drive.

This built-in motivation remains strong as people age.

There appears to be a link between engagement in meaningful activity and well-being, which relates to the needs of people with dementia.

People with dementia seem to be at risk of not 'doing,' which can lead to ill-being. (Why do we think this might be?)

They can help people maintain their skills and give them a sense of achievement.

They can provide interest or fun and help the person feel better about themselves and be more alert and interested in what is

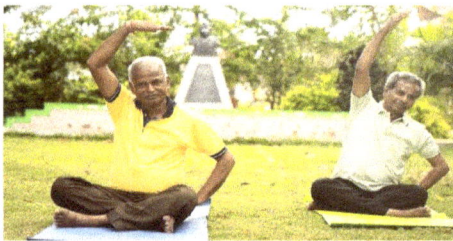

happening around them.

Activities such as painting a picture or looking at old photographs may help people with dementia express their feelings, so be sensitive to their reactions.

What Activities Can You Do?

- Write down a list of five everyday activities you have done on the last day.
- Does your list include a mixture of leisure, work, and self-care activities, providing a balanced lifestyle?
- Do these activities help you to maintain your skills and provide exercise and mental stimulation?
- Do these activities allow you choice, independence, a sense of worth, self-esteem, social inclusion, and a sense of purpose?
- How do you think your balance of activities and the benefits you get from them compared with those in your residents' lives?

Here are a few activities you can choose from:

Exercise: Exercising in the fresh air daily is enjoyable and a healthy form of physical activity. The patient can also exercise with music, which often helps improve people's moods. For example, if they like dancing, they can designate a space for it and dance to their favourite melodies. Moreover, games such as playing with a ball or balloon can help make exercise fun if approached lightheartedly.

Walking is essential for people with dementia to keep them mentally and physically fit. While walking, they can grab a friend, enjoy a cup of coffee, and visit a café, garden centre, or local museum. It will also help build connections with others and provide a change of scene and a focal point for conversation.

Music: Even listening to music can help improve mood. A carer or family member can record some favourite pieces, especially familiar songs from the patient's younger days. They may like to sing along with the words, or you may want to sing together.

Pets: Many people with dementia respond well to pets, especially if they had a pet earlier. If you do not have a pet, you can encourage a friend or neighbour to bring one in from time to time.

Television: Television can become increasingly confusing as dementia progresses. If a dementia patient enjoys watching television, try to select some favourite programs and still follow rather   than   have   them   on   all   day.

Why Are They Important at the Early Stage of Dementia?

People at an early stage may place greater significance on typical everyday activities to maintain a sense of continuity and contribution.

The person can plan to work towards achieving a goal but may need direction.

Directions need to be simple.

The person may be able to carry out familiar tasks in familiar surroundings.

Why Are They Important at Moderate Stage of Dementia?

They are more likely to participate in activities they can relate to, such as reminiscing about a time they can recall.

Participation is more concerned with the process of taking part than the result.

The person is experiencing growing difficulties in perceiving and understanding the world of 'others.'

Sequencing a task is impaired, and more complex activities must be directed one step at a time.

Why are They Important at the Later stage of Dementia?

Movement is a reflex response to the stimulus.

Direct stimulation raises a person's self-awareness.

A warm and reassuring tone and voice volume are vital to establishing rapport.

Use Primitive reflexes - smiling, waving, handshake.

Responses to Activities

Observe the person responding to the activity.

If the person appears uncomfortable or distressed, do not continue the activity.

If the person seems upset, try to analyse why this may have occurred.

Communication is the Key

Communication with dementia patients is challenging and must be different. For example, they can easily pick up on negative body language, such as sighs and raised eyebrows, which will affect their behaviour.

Therefore, there are some general rules regarding communicating with a dementia patient. Firstly, the person is dementing, not demented, which means that many mental functions remain relatively intact until the later stages of illness. Therefore, keep these retained abilities in practice as much as possible.

Another common mistake that carers and others make is talking down to the person as if they were a child or not present. This kind of approach is both demeaning and might provoke resentment. So, try to talk like you would usually on an adult-adult level, but keep things simple. For example, you can say shorter sentences with only one subject to make it easier for the patient to understand.

Moreover, when asking questions, avoid the 'multiple choice' approach. For example, instead of asking, 'Would you like to go out for a dinner or movie or concert?', it would be better to break down the question into two or three parts. Use gestures, and speak clearly and slowly but avoid being overly formal.

Give them time to respond and leave space in the conversation. Then, allow them to initiate and lead the discussion.

It would be best if you used person-centric dementia language as it will help to promote dementia-friendly communities.

You can also use the 'ABC approach' to help when talking with someone experiencing difficulties in using language or engaging in conversation.

Avoid Confrontation

Be Practical

Clarify the feeling and comfort!

DO	DON'T
Speak to the person in a tone that conveys respect and dignity.	For example, talk to the person in 'baby talk' or as if you are talking to a child.
Keep your explanations short. Use clear and flexible language.	Use complicated words or phrases and long sentences.
Maintain eye contact by positioning yourself at the person's eye level.	Glare at, or 'eyeball', the person you are talking to.
Look directly at the person and ensure that you have their attention before you speak. Always begin by identifying yourself and explaining what you propose to do.	Begin a task without explaining who you are or what you are about to do. Talk to the person without eye contact, such as while rummaging in a drawer to select clothing.
Use visual cues whenever possible.	Try and compete in a distracting environment.
Be realistic in expectations.	Provoke a fatal reaction through unrealistic expectations or by asking the person to do more than

	one task at a time.
Observe and attempt to interpret a person's non-verbal communication.	Disregard your non-verbal communication.
Paraphrase and use a calm and reassuring tone of voice.	Disregard talk that may seem to be 'rambling.'
Speak slowly and say individual words clearly. Use strategies to reduce the effects of hearing impairment.	Shout or talk too fast.
Encourage talk about things that they are familiar with.	Interrupt only if it can be helped.
Use touch if appropriate.	Attempt to touch or invade their personal space if they show signs of fear or aggression.

Dementia and Language

One of the early signs of dementia is not finding the right words, especially people and objects' names. The person may use an incorrect word or need help finding a word. During the later stages, the patient may reach a point where they can hardly communicate through language. Besides using incorrect words, they may completely forget the names of objects or people.

Moreover, they may confuse relations and generations, such as mistaking their child for their nephew or their wife for their mother. This may undoubtedly be distressing for their loved ones, but it's a part of their memory loss.

Since the brain starts processing the information incorrectly, the person with dementia may be trying to interpret a world that no longer makes sense to them; they may talk about objects or people they have never seen.

A crucial part of dementia is when individuals and those around them start misinterpreting each other's communication. These misunderstandings can be problematic and may require some support and technique to deal with them. This can be frustrating and upsetting for the person with dementia and those around them. However, there are several ways to ensure that you understand each other.

Tips: Communicating with a Person Having Dementia

General Advice

- Listen carefully to what the person has to say.
- Make sure the person is fully attentive before you speak.
- Speak clearly.
- Use physical contact to reassure the person.
- Pay attention to body language.
- Be patient and respectful; remember, it may take longer for the brain to process the information and respond.
- Consider how things appear in the reality of the person with dementia.
- Determine if any other factors are affecting communication.

Listening Skills

- Be attentive while listening to what the person is saying, and keep encouraging them.
- If the person feels sad, let them express their feelings without trying to lighten up their mood forcefully. Sometimes the person needs to vent out and get reassurance.
- If the person needs help finishing a sentence or finding the right word, ask them to explain differently. Again, listen out for clues and try making sense of their sentences.
- If you find the speech hard to understand, use what you know about the person to interpret what they might be trying to say. But always recheck to ensure you are right-it's infuriating to have your sentence finished incorrectly by someone else!

Attract the Person's Attention

- Try to grab the attention of the person before you start to communicate.
- Make eye contact, as it will help them focus on you.

- Make sure they can see you.
- Try to minimise surrounding noises, such as TV, radio, or other people's conversation.

Use Body Language

- Never stand over someone to communicate, as it can feel intimidating. Instead, drop below your eye level. It will help them feel more in control of the situation.
- Stay close to the person, as it can also feel intimidating. Always respect their personal space.
- Stay calm, focused, and still while you communicate. This shows the person that you give them your full attention and that you have time for them.
- Keep yourself relaxed and keep your body language normal as a person with dementia can read your body language. Therefore, a worried facial expression or agitated movements may distress or upset them, making communication more difficult.
- If the person cannot communicate appropriately, pick up cues from their body language. The way they move about and hold themselves and the expression on their face can give you clear signals about how they are feeling.

Speak Clearly

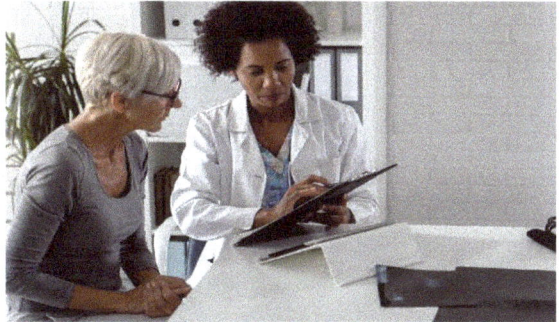

- As dementia progresses, the person will become less able to start a conversation, so you may have to start taking the initiative.
- If the person needs help understanding what you are saying, try saying it differently instead of merely repeating the same thing.
- Try to lighten up the atmosphere with humour whenever you can. It can help to bring you closer together. So, try

to laugh together about mistakes and misunderstandings- it can help.
- Speak calmly and clearly. Avoid raising your voice or speaking sharply, as this may distress the person even if they cannot follow the sense of your words.

Use short and simple sentences.

- Avoid asking direct questions. People with dementia can become annoyed if they can't find the answer and may respond with aggression or irritation. So, ask questions one at a time and phrase them in a way that allows for a 'yes' or 'no' answer.
- Try to avoid asking the person to make complicated decisions. Too many choices can become confusing and frustrating.
- Allow enough time for the person to process information as it will take longer than it used to. They may feel pressured if you try to hurry.

What/Who is Reality?

- Facts and fantasy can become confusing with each stage of dementia. If someone says something you know isn't right, don't respond with a direct no or contradict them. Instead, try to find ways around the situation.
- If the person says, 'We should go now- Mother is waiting for me,' you might reply, 'Your mother used to wait for you, didn't she?'
- Avoid making the person with dementia feel foolish in front of other people by contradicting their statements or replying to the above sentence with, 'Your mother is dead. '

Physical Contact

- Even when the conversation becomes more complex, being affectionate or warm can help carers remain close to their loved ones or for the person with dementia to feel supported.
- Communicate your affection or care by the touch of your hand and the tone of your voice.
- Try to provide reassurance by patting or holding the person's hand or putting your arm around them if it feels right.
- Show Respect
- Ensure no one treats the person with dementia like a child or speaks down to them, even if they don't understand what people say.
- Try to include the person in conversations with others and have them in social groups. It can help a person with dementia preserve their identity's fragile sense. It also helps to protect them from overwhelming feelings of isolation and exclusion.
- If you get little response from the person, you can try to speak about the person as if they weren't there. But don't disregard them in a way that can make them feel frustrated and cut off.

Other   Causes   of   Communication   Difficulties
It is vital to remember that communication can be affected by other factors apart from dementia- for example:

If you suspect illness, discomfort, pain, or the side effects of medication, talk to the person's doctor or GP.

Problems may occur with hearing, sight, or ill-fitting dentures. Please ensure the person's glasses are according to their current eye-sight number, their hearing aids are working correctly, and their dentures are well-fitted and comfortable.

(H) Assistive Technologies for Help

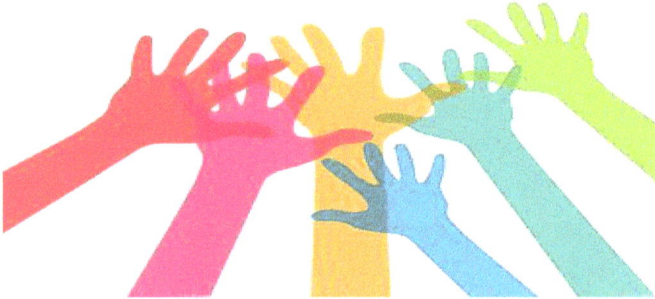

What is Assistive Technology?

Assistive technology refers to devices or systems that help improve or maintain a person's ability, independence, and self-being by assisting them to do things in everyday life. These can 'assist' with a range of difficulties, including problems with memory and mobility.

Some are specially designed to assist with cognitive and physical functions associated with dementia, such as electronic pillboxes (that remind you to take medication on time) to 'smart home' systems (that you can instruct to switch off the lights or turn up the heating). Others are regular products that can help everyone. It also includes various applications in smartphones and tablets, specifically developed for people with dementia.

However, over time the apps dedicated to general use may replace some initially developed products for people with dementia. For example, electronic medication alarms could be replaced by smartphone calendar apps.

Even though I have listed some fantastic devices that can assist you or your loved one in living a better quality of life, here are some commonly used ones:

✓ Bed sensor alarm
✓ Chair sensor alarm
✓ Baby monitors
✓ Pendant alarms
✓ Clocks with day and date

This technology can help with everyday tasks and activities, improve your safety, monitor your health, or help people support you. Assistive technology is best for people for the following purposes:

✓ communication, including speech
✓ hearing and sight
✓ keeping you safe both inside and outside the home
✓ maintaining self-confidence and independence
✓ memory and understanding of problems
✓ safe mobility
✓ problems with planning and carrying out daily activities.
✓ socialising and doing things you enjoy

How Can Assistive Technology Help Dementia Sufferers?

The way assistive technology can be used to assist a dementia patient varies greatly. It ranges from simple, standalone devices to complex, integrated systems that help a person be independent for as long as possible. Patients can use any of these devices, depending on the stage of dementia.

A few areas where assistive technology may help include everyday living, safety, monitoring, communication, and prompts and reminders.

1. Safety
   Assistive technology for dementia patients primarily provides safety and security. For example, motion sensor technology at home can prevent falls and injuries by silently alerting carers when patients with a high risk of falling move away from their beds or chair.

2. Everyday Tasks

Assistive technology can also support dementia patients in carrying out everyday tasks. For this purpose, may include devices and equipment like automated ovens, dishwashers and washing machines, lamp and light activation, electronic showers, taps and toilets, floor cleaning robots, automatic window and curtain controls, garden sensors for automated watering, and temperature sensors for automatic climate control.

Point-of-care technologies also help dementia patients living alone in their early stages or without a carer. It can monitor a person's daily health condition, such as blood pressure, blood sugar, and heart rate. This data can be automatically transferred to the health professional, who can monitor vital signs and make appropriate decisions about required interventions.

3.Communication

Instead of providing round-the-clock, one-on-one supervision, assistive technology can simplify communication and assistance between carers, patients, and their family members. For example, video conferencing facilitates communication with health professionals and service providers. This is especially important when the patient resides at a significant distance from the health clinic. In such cases, assistive technology helps relieve the pressure on carers and supports their efforts in delivering care in the best possible manner.

Moreover, online communication can also help dementia patients not feel lonely or isolated. They can communicate with their friends and family and participate in significant family events through networked computers with internet capabilities. Access to online browsing, research, learning, and games can also help broaden a person's interests.

4. Monitoring

In cases where a person with dementia is prone to disorientation and wandering, assistive technology such as virtual door and exit sensors that detect entry and exit can alert family members and carers. Moreover, GPS tracking devices can also monitor the person's exact location within meters.

5. Prompts and Reminders

Assistive technology also includes unique solutions that can positively impact the health and well-being of dementia patients. For example, automatic medication dispensers help dementia patients maintain medication compliance, orientation clocks help with confusion about the time, day of the week, month, or year, and locator devices allow one to find lost items.

Benefits of Assistive Technology

It's imperative to understand that assistive technology is not about technology. Instead, it is about improving a person's quality of life through improved living standards, greater independence, safeguarding, and social interaction.
Some of the critical benefits of assistive technology include the following:

- ✓ increased choice, independence, safety, and sense of control
- ✓ improved quality of life
- ✓ improved support for people with long-term health conditions
- ✓ maintenance of the ability to remain at home.
- ✓ the reduced burden placed on carers.
- ✓ reduced falls and accidents at home

Types of Devices

Look at some assistive technologies that can help make the life of dementia patients much more comfortable.

1. Universal TV Remote Control

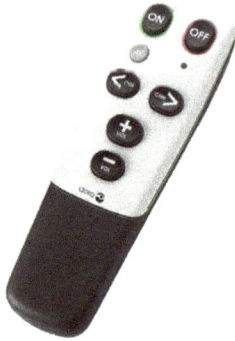

Doro Handle Easy 321rc is specially designed for people who want an easy remote control. Change channels and adjust your TV or radio volume with seven programmable remote keys.

Easy-to-press buttons

Easy to understand.

Oversized button

2. Doorphone Video Intercom with Monitor

• Wired video intercom giving you a view of who is at the door

• 4 meters night vision giving you the ability to see at all hours

(Images are only to make you understand better, check references at the end of the book)

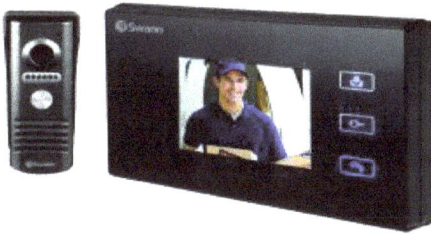

3. **Red Handled Cutlery**

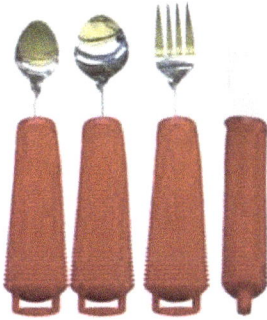

This cutlery set is easy to use and helps people with restricted hand/wrist movements or visual and memory problems. Mealtime can be more enjoyable with this easy-to-grip and latex-free cutlery set, which features bendable stainless steel shafts to help you quickly use each piece.

4. **Medelert One Month Pill Dispenser**

Modelert is a fully automatic, lockable lid and timed release of medication.

(Images are only to make you understand better, check references at the end of the book)

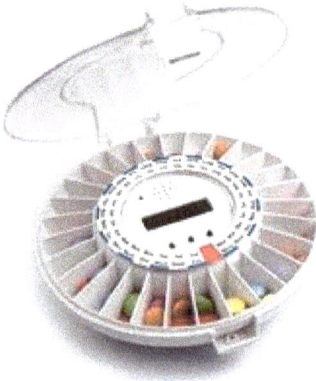

5. Pill Dispenser Medelert

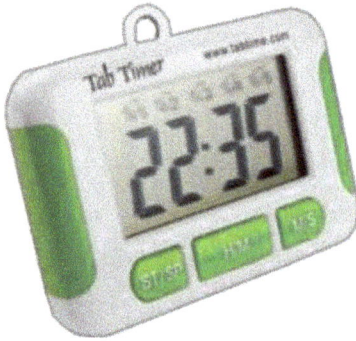

Up to 5 daily alarms at whatever times are required.

6. Pill Daily Reminder

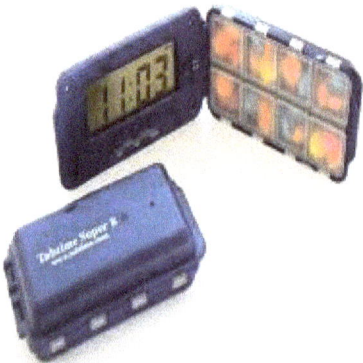

PILL TIMER SUPER 8

Up to 8 daily alarms at whatever times you require.

(Images are only to make you understand better, check references at the end of the book)

7. Black Wallet Pill Organizer

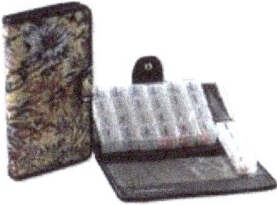

Daily & weekly pill & tablet organiser with luxurious 'chamois leather' effect

8. Doro Secure Mobile 58

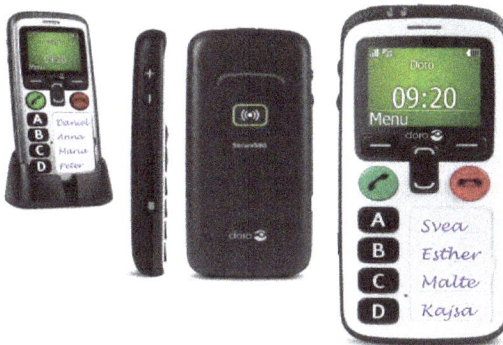

Durable and splash-proof (IP54) mobile phone with four-speed dial keys for calling people you rely on with a straightforward press. Feel even safer thanks to an assistance button and a safety timer that can automatically dial up and send an SMS alarm to pre-set numbers, along with GPS localisation to let people know where you are. In addition, contacts can be managed by a trusted relative over the internet using the Doro Experience Manager.

Great safety functions

GPS localisation

Speakerphone

9. Geolocation Phone

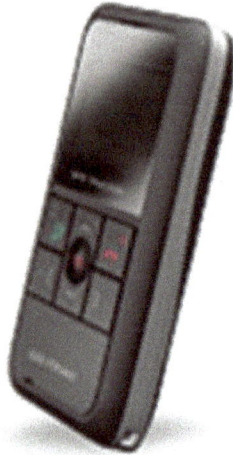

Geolocation Phone is part of a system specially designed for people requiring support and constant monitoring. It is easy to use a phone with a speed dial and SOS functionality. Importantly it contains GPS/GPRS tracking allowing the device's location to be monitored within 2 meters. Real-time tracking, movement, and impact sensors combined with 'Geo-Fencing' enable and alert the monitoring service when the device moves, has been shocked or has left a pre-defined safe zone. The unique combination of technology provides a small, powerful device enabling a world-class monitoring solution.

(Images are only to make you understand better, check references at the end of the book)

10. Personal Tracker Phone

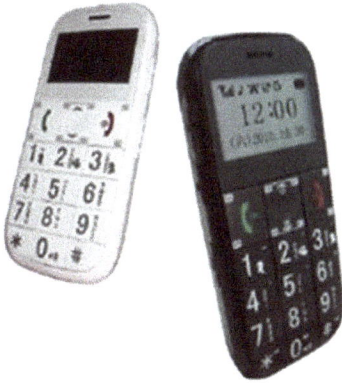

Dual Tracking Options Gsm/GPRS

Extra-Large Keypad Buttons - Extra Large Text

It Can Track Complete Journeys with Location History Detailed on the Website or Can Send Location Coordinates with Google Mapping Link to Authorized Mobile Phones (Up To 3)

11. Peephole Camera

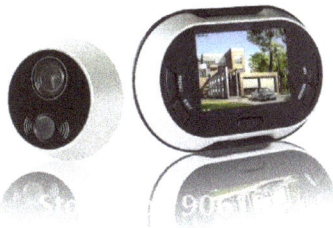

Better visibility of big images: the digital door viewer can neatly and clearly show images, unlike traditional door viewers, which distort images.

Both children who are not tall enough and the with poorer eyesight aged can easily see people outside the doors.

Digital 3.5-inch LCD Video Door Viewer Peephole Doorbell Security Camera

12. Intruder/Inactivity Monitoring using PIR Detection

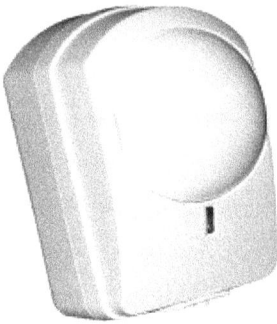

Inactivity Monitor

The PIR can look for movement within a defined time. If the user has not moved within that period, for example, due to a fall or feeling unwell, the care phone will send an alarm to the carer/monitoring centre.

Intruder Monitoring

If the user leaves their property to stay with friends or visit a day centre, pressing a button on the care phone and the portable button will set the system into 'away' mode, providing a basic intruder alarm system for the property.

(Images are only to make you understand better, check references at the end of the book)

Digital Desktop Clock

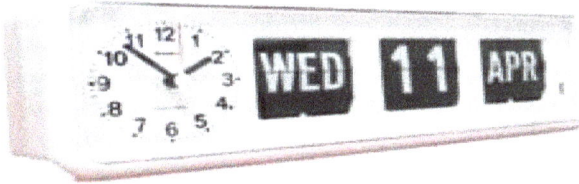

It is a new variation of a clock used in care homes. These clocks are massively popular among those who find it challenging to keep track of the days and months. Particularly useful for Assisted Living and those who have Alzheimer's and Dementia. A unique feature of the clock is that it requires no adjustment at the end of the calendar month. This is called a Perpetual Calendar System. The clock will even take care of the leap years for you, again requiring no intervention from the end user.

Many cheaper models will not offer you this automation, and you will need to mess around changing back and forth for long and short months. Not so here. It should be noted that these clocks DO need an initial set-up and will not automatically be set to the correct time when you first put the batteries in. However, it is a short process with complete instructions on the back of the clock (so you can keep them). The only adjustments needed for the clock's running will be when summer and winter change. After that, the process will be quick.

13. Adapted Crockery Set

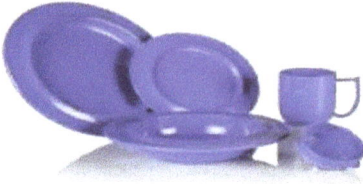

As dementia progresses, eating can be more challenging as coordination declines, and it becomes harder to feed yourself using standard crockery and cutlery. Swallowing and chewing can also get more difficult in the later stages of dementia. This can mean eating a meal takes longer, and food is more likely to go cold, making the whole experience less enjoyable.

This Find adaptive crockery set is made from hard-wearing melamine, which means it's less likely to shatter if dropped, is dishwasher safe, and is lightweight, so it's easier for people with less strength to use.

The plates and cups have a broad base for greater stability, while a lipped rim reduces spillages. This can help improve the manipulation of food and ultimately maintain someone's dignity while eating- a key component for a good quality of life.

The set includes two plates (7" x 10"), a dish, and a cup with a lid.

(Images are only to make you understand better, check references at the end of the book)

14. Big Digit Talking Watch

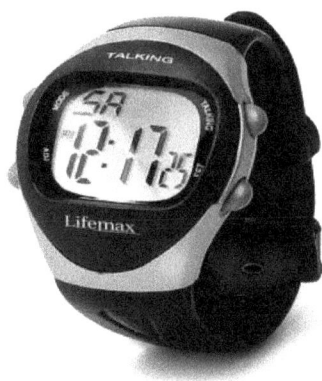

(Images are only to make you understand better, check references at the end of the book)

With large LCD digits, this watch also shows the time and date and speaks to them.

Great as a sports watch with a talking stopwatch feature, this watch is designed with optional hourly time announcements and four alarms to act as helpful reminders. Incredibly useful if you take medication up to 4 times a day.

15. Bed and Chair Leaving Alarms

The wide selection of Bed, Chair, and Floor alarms will alert you if a loved one tries to get out of their bed, chair, or leave the room. The standalone alarms can alarm locally or be connected to a service provider. So, no matter where you are in the house, you will be notified.

120 Alarm & Mat Alarm Power Supply

Long Term Bed Pad for Double Bed

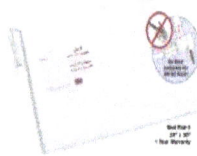

Pager With Fall Alarm Interface

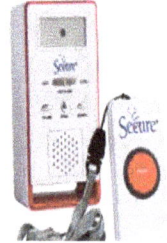

Secure Controller PSU

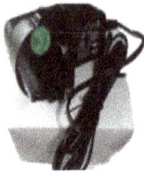

Universal Bed Leaving Alarm Kit

Bed Alarm and Pager Kit. If someone leaves the bed the pager alarms

Replacement Bed Pad

Bed Mat and Pager Kit

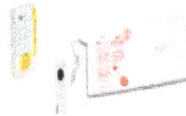

120 Bed and Chair Alarm

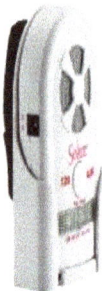

120 Floor Mat Alarm

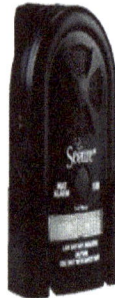

Universal Bed & Chair Alarm

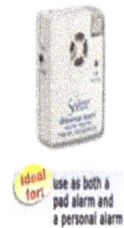

16. Digital Dementia Clock

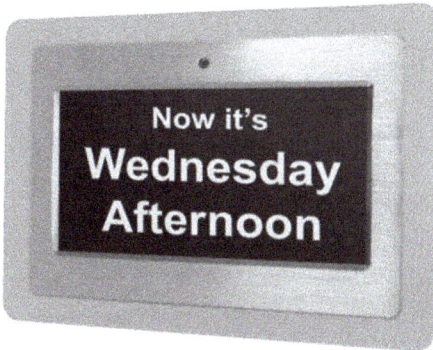

The design features a straightforward display showing the time of day as either morning, afternoon, evening, or night. The Dementia Day Clock is ideal for people living with dementia as they can lose the ability to distinguish between day and night. Therefore, Alzheimer's Day Clock can assist primary carers by ensuring a daily routine can be maintained.

17. KEY SAFE C500

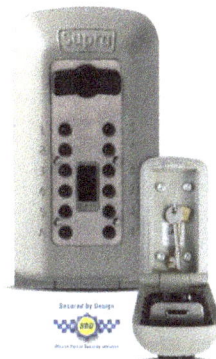

(Images are only to make you understand better, check references at the end of the book)

The Supra C500 KeySafe was designed after extensive consultation with users.

18. Care Unity Main Unit

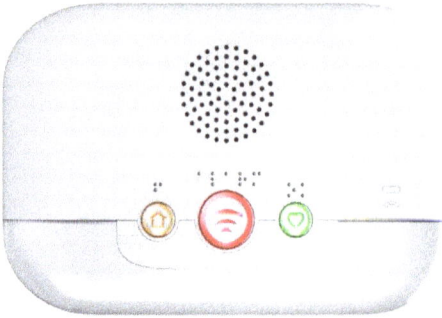

This stylishly designed all-in-one CareUnity unit is in crisp white and black to complement all home interiors. In addition, the Braille button identifiers for visually impaired users allow care monitoring to match evolving care needs precisely.

CareUnity meets people's needs across every part of the care spectrum, either in their own home or a formal care setting – from those requiring only the most basic safety monitoring to customers with more complex care needs, including dementia and fall management.

19. Wrist-Worn Fall Detector

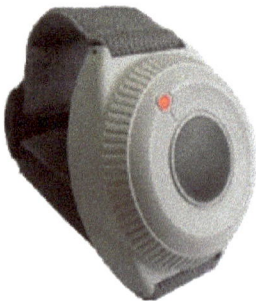

(Images are only to make you understand better, check references at the end of the book)

The wrist-worn fall detector provides a more discreet way of wearing a fall trigger with an integral alarm button, so a different pendant is not required. It uses technology to calculate its position as the person wearing it moves around before a fall.

When a fall alarm is raised, the technology allows a small period to verify that the fall is real. The device has two settings whereby the self-cancellation period can be left on or turned off for a quicker response. If the self-cancellation is left on the device, the device will vibrate 26 times. The call will be cancelled if movement is detected in this period. The fall detector is hypoallergenic and waterproof.

Memory Clinics

With advanced stages, memory can become a significant issue for dementia patients. Therefore, I recommend that dementia patients visit memory clinics to improve their quality of life, which is highly affected by poor memory.

Do you need to learn what a memory clinic is? Then, let's learn about it below.

What is a Memory Clinic?

Memory Clinics are independent clinics primarily aimed at improving practice in identifying, investigating, and treating memory disorders, including dementia. Staff employed at Memory Clinics are specially trained to diagnose memory problems and provide people concerned about cognitive and memory problems with a diagnosis, information, treatment (when necessary), and advice.

People from various countries with dementia have never had a formal diagnosis. Therefore, it has been identified that early diagnosis of Alzheimer's Disease or any related dementias is critical to acquiring appropriate treatments, managing financial and legal affairs (including getting a Power of Attorney), and accessing support services.

Moreover, early diagnosis also helps the person experiencing the symptoms to be more proactive in lifestyle decision-making and planning their future-care options. Once a diagnosis is made, treatment can also be initiated by Memory Clinic staff, and advice can be given on anything, including memory aids, banking, driving, employment, family matters, and leisure time interests. Memory Clinics may also provide post-diagnostic counselling and emotional support for newly diagnosed people.

How to Avail Memory Clinic Services?

Anyone can avail of the services of a Memory Clinic. However, most clinics only accept referrals from GPs or other healthcare workers. Therefore, if you have noticed that your memory is not as sharp as before and are worried about it, you should discuss it with your GP.

They will analyze if there's a significant issue after a series of tests and making a diagnosis of dementia. Or the GP may decide that further in-depth assessment is required and may refer you to a Memory Clinic.

What Information Will Clients and Their Family Members be asked at The Memory Clinic Assessment?

Taking a family member or a close friend during your visit to a Memory Clinic is recommended. This is because the latter can, if necessary, provide staff with additional information regarding the person's memory and cognitive problems and overall health.

During the clinic appointment, a series of questions will be asked by the clinic staff of the person referred to the clinic. Additional questions will also be asked regarding the family member, where appropriate.

The information sought during the appointment includes the following:

- ✓ the person's general health
- ✓ signs and symptoms of memory problems
- ✓ risk factors for Alzheimer's disease and related dementias such as smoking, obesity, diabetes, family history, and blood pressure
- ✓ behavioural/personality changes
- ✓ educational attainments and literacy level
- ✓ physical functioning and activities of daily living.

Neuropsychological assessment/testing may also occur, which usually involves a series of questions assessing short-term and long-term memory, language, orientation, attention, perception, and calculation. The latter can be brief or more in-depth.

Do All People Who Visit a Memory Clinic Receive a Diagnosis?

Generally, everybody who attends a Memory Clinic receives feedback on the results of the formal assessment. For example, these results may show that there is no organic memory problem, although the person has a subjective memory complaint, or that the person has a Mild Cognitive Impairment (MCI) - a condition which is not a normal part of ageing, and which is characterised by significant cognitive impairment in the absence of dementia - or that the person has dementia.

If a clinical diagnosis is established, it is discussed with the person if they wish. However, it is generally recommended that clinic staff consult the person's diagnosis if there are clear reasons against doing this.

However, an important point to note is that Memory Clinics may not be suitable for assessing all cases of dementia. They are more useful in suspected early dementia and patients with no significant associated psychological or medical problems.

An aged care assessment team and a geriatrician can better assess frail older people and those with more severe cognitive impairment. Similarly, senior care mental health services would help determine psychotic or depressed people with suspected dementia.

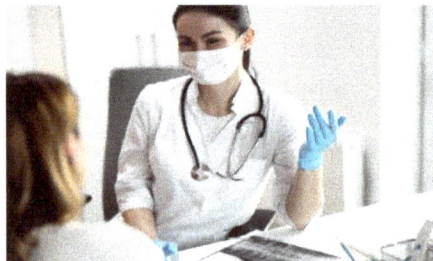

Assessments by these various other services will include many multidisciplinary evaluations (discussed in Chapter E) in memory clinics. However, they are different for everyone; they are tailored to individual cases. For example, many people with mild dementia, and most with moderate to severe dementia, will not require a neuropsychological examination.

What Is Information Given to People Worried About Their Memory and Those Diagnosed with MCI Or Dementia?

Extensive information is provided to people who attend Memory Clinics. The type of information supplied typically includes:

- Advice about continuing or not continuing to drive.
- Advice about continuing or not continuing to work.
- Clarification of memory problem symptoms
- Diagnosis, including differential diagnosis
- General tips for dealing with memory problems.
- Leisure time activities
- Treatment information, such as advice about anti-dementia drugs and how they work
- Ways to improve and maintain cognitive health.

What Treatments and Services Are Offered at Memory Clinics?

Treatments and services offered at Memory Clinics vary according to each person's individual needs. These treatments are usually classified as pharmacological (drugs) or non-pharmacological (no drugs).

In some cases, pharmacological interventions such as anti-dementia drugs (cholinesterase inhibitors) are offered to people with early dementia or Mild Cognitive Impairment. These drugs help to slow down memory loss or the rate of progression of dementia. However, it should be noted that the drugs are not curative and do not tackle the condition's underlying cause.

Even though anti-dementia drugs can be effective in the short term, they unfortunately only work in one-third of all cases. A different type of medicine called Memantine is sometimes offered to people with more advanced dementia.

Non-pharmacological interventions are also often offered through most Memory Clinic services. They include counselling, information, advice on practical everyday aids designed to improve quality of life, and recommendations about relaxation therapies and ways to help reduce challenging behaviours.

Other Referrals to Consider

Fortunately, many organisations, assistive centres, and societies always lend a helping hand to people who have dementia and their families.
Old Age Psychiatry

Occupational Therapy

Speech and Language Therapy

Essential Tips to Keep the Brain Healthy

Stay Physically Active

Thirty minutes of exercise five times weekly can also help your brain stay fit.

Stay Mentally Active

Activities that make you think and concentrate, like doing crosswords and Sudoku, help your brain stay healthy.

Learn New Things

Learning or doing new things like reading, art, music, and theatre helps strengthen your brain.

Meet People

Meeting family and friends, especially out and about, helps protect your brain from slowing down and enables you to live longer.

Reduce Stress

Stress is terrible for your brain and your memory. Relaxing and not worrying helps your brain work well.

Sleep Well

Sleep is essential for our brains to work typically. So make sure you are comfortable at night and allow yourself to rest.

Eat a Good Diet

Good food helps to protect your brain. Eat foods like fruit, dark vegetables and fish. Try to avoid alcohol and smoking.

Think Positive

Think young and be positive. Focus on what you CAN do!

(I) Dementia-Friendly Designs

What is Dementia Friendly Design?

The design of a home or building that enables and supports everyone regardless of size, age, size, disability, or ability and at the same time is usable, accessible, and easily understood by people with dementia is a complex task.

Design Issues for a UD Design Approach

Consider the following eight design issues as part of a UD (Universal Design) approach for dementia-friendly homes:

> Encourage participation and discussion by dementia patients, their families, and carers in the design finalisation.
> Use familiar design with recognizable features consistent with user expectations.
> Support personalisation of the environment to enhance continuity of self.
> Provide an environment that is easy to interpret and calm, paying close attention to reducing acoustic and visual disturbances.
> Provide good visual access to critical areas of the dwelling or important objects to remind and prompt the occupant when required.
> Provide unobtrusive safety measures and appropriate technology such as Assistive Technology (AT), Ambient Assisted Living (AAL), Telecare, or Telehealth to provide a safe and secure environment.
> Create distinct spaces for domestic activities to make their meaning and function more memorable and legible.
> Provide accessible and safe outdoor spaces perceptible from the interior to encourage occupant use of these spaces.

These issues must be carefully managed to ensure a balanced

design approach for UD dementia-friendly dwellings. Considering these issues within the UD framework will ensure that the home meets the specific needs of people with dementia while supporting other occupants, family members, or carers.

Some Commonly Used UD Dementia-Friendly Features

Some Typical UD Dementia-Friendly Features

> Ensure the right acoustic conditions by orientating spaces away from noise sources or providing high acoustic insulation levels such as triple glazing.
> Create a separate entrance by planting shrubs or providing different colours to the entrance area or front gate.
> Provide level entry front and back doors.
> Provide a brightly painted front door to make it distinct and recognisable.
> Consider fitting a curtain to cover the inside of the door. This discourages a person with dementia from leaving the house at inappropriate times if necessary.
> Ensure window dressing, such as curtains or blinds, does not obscure natural light and provides maximum views of the exterior or vital external features.
> Avoid strong patterns for floor finishes and provide plain-coloured, matt finishes that reduce glare or shine in brightly lit conditions.
> Provide a continuous floor finish with as little change in material as possible. If it is essential to change the material, ensure minimum colour contrast, particularly at door thresholds.
> Use a contrasting door colour to ensure that the door is easily distinguished from the surrounding walls.
> Use contrasting colours on the skirting boards to provide a visual break between the walls and the floors to ensure greater visual contrast.

➢ Ensure that window location, sill height, and dressing facilitate visual access to safe external areas or objects, such as a dustbin or clothesline.

➢ Consider using glazed kitchen units or cupboards to provide visual access to the contents.

➢ Ensure easy and, where possible, level access to safe and accessible outdoor space to encourage a person to spend time outside or engage in outdoor activities.

➢ Provide critical objects such as recycling bins or clotheslines within view and easy reach to maximise independence and encourage typical daily household activities.

➢ Provide a distinctive colour to the entry doors of the main rooms, such as the bathroom.

➢ Ensure proper artificial lighting is provided in circulation areas, especially those leading to toilets and bathrooms that might be used at night.

➢ Provide colour contrast between the floor and the steps to highlight the presence of the stairs.

➢ Ensure that the handrail stands out from the wall, for example, by painting it a different colour.

➢ Provide visual access to the wardrobe, and where appropriate, consider a glazed section to the closet to enable a person to see their clothes hanging inside to facilitate dressing.

Considerations When Designing for Dementia Care

With the projected rise in dementia cases worldwide, I believe the number of facilities equipped to help people suffering from this condition will increase to meet the demand. In addition, these facilities will allow a better quality of residential care and independent living for residents with various illnesses and levels of dementia.

Therefore, they must ensure that older people are given ultimate care, which helps them feel at home and are kept secure and safe. This requires considered interior design and a careful selection of interior finishes.

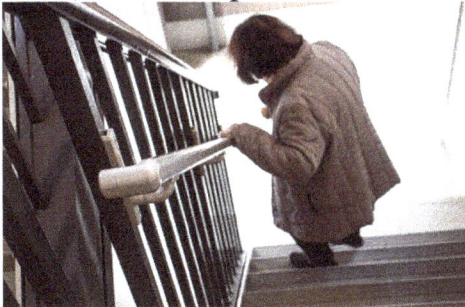

Fortunately, a wide range of high-performance products on the market can create comfortable, welcoming, and stress-free environments without compromising resident safety or hygiene, reducing whole-life costs and maintenance.

I have come across so many dementia patients and the difficulties they must face at home or in dementia care. The following considerations will certainly help improve their quality of life.

Understand the Patient's Requirements

The first step in designing a facility for dementia patients is to consider their state of mind, condition, and how they can help them.

Since dementia affects cognitive functionality and memory, often resulting in confusion and misinterpretations, choosing the right colours and textures when designing the facility is crucial. For example, patients might misinterpret a change in floor colour as a step.

Such confusion may make a person with dementia feel scared and disoriented. Therefore, keeping such perceptions and impairments in mind when designing a space and choosing wall and floor finishes is critical.

Make the Essential Things Prominent

Another critical point to consider is making essential things stand out, using colours, and designing unimportant ones that do not make the area or things prominent. This includes things like doors and handrails.

Distinctive and bold colours can highlight the areas the patients should use or notice, such as handrails and doorways. Bars will also give them physical and psychological support, so they won't fall, making them feel confident and secure.

Another good idea is to be tactful while playing with colours. For example, the same-coloured walls and doors can prevent the patient from entering inaccessible areas, such as plant areas or staff offices, as the same colour won't let the door stand out.

Long-Lasting and Inexpensive Designs

Even though many people with dementia require wheelchairs or walking aids, the wall and floor furnishing should still look good so that the look doesn't seem very institutional or clinical. This will enable them to feel more at home and comfortable.

Impact-resistant panel systems and wall protection sheets are great for inexpensively creating a stable welcoming environment. They are also easy to clean and are strong enough to cope with daily wear and tear.

These products come in an array of colours and finishes to help minimise the institutional feel of a space and, in some cases, feature artwork or photos, turning an image into a protective surface.

Eliminate Wandering and Getting Lost

As dementia progresses, the patients often feel the urge to wander about and usually forget where they are going or how to get back.

For this reason, many dementia units have been designed in recent years to enable 'wandering with a purpose,' providing patients with a destination or somewhere to focus. So, for example, there can be a communal area or a library set up at the end of the corridor to give residents a place to wander or walk. This will encourage them to move around independently without the fear of getting lost.

Use the Reminiscence Therapy

Today, reminiscence therapy is one of the leading therapeutic approaches in dementia care, helping patients communicate with their carers and other patients.

As discussed before, dementia primarily affects short-term memory, which is what his therapy caters to dementia patients. However, it enables them to use their long-term memory and recall stories from their past. According to Martina Kane of the Alzheimer's Society, the main advantage of reminiscence therapy is "...that it's person-centred, it can be very individualized," It also helps the carers to get to know their patients personally from other angles apart from the disease.

A design trend that helps in reminiscence therapy is using imagery on interior doors and walls. It has had positive results in mental health environments and dementia care. However, this imagery is wider than signage; it also involves printing.

Since nature elements are highly effective at reducing stress and promoting wellness, parts of walls can feature local scenery, such as sea views, woodlands, and historical images of the local area. They will be a positive distraction and take the patients down their memory lanes- back to a time or place they knew while facilitating the reminiscing process.

References

"5 Considerations When Designing for Dementia Care." n.d. *Construction Specialists*. Document. 17 February 2021.

https://www.c-sgroup.co.uk/blog/5-considerations-when-designing-for-dementia-care/

Access. n.d. 10 February 2021.

https://www.theaccessgroup.com/blog/assistive-technology-improve-dementia-care/?navtype=v2

"AD8 Dementia Screening Interview." 2005. *alz.org*. 28 January 2021.

https://www.alz.org/media/Documents/ad8-dementia-screening.pdf

Alzheimer Europe. 8 October 2009. Document. 28 January 2021.

https://www.alzheimer-europe.org/

Alzheimer's Society. n.d. 10 February 2021.

https://www.theaccessgroup.com/blog/assistive-technology-improve-dementia-care/?navtype=v2

Alzheimer's Society UK (United Against Dementia). n.d. Document. 17 February 2021.

https://www.alzheimers.org.uk/

"Chapter 1 - What is Dementia?" *Dementia: Ethical issues*. UK, 2014.

https://www.nuffieldbioethics.org/wp-content/uploads/2014/07/Chapter-1-What-is-dementia1.pdf

"Communicating." August 2020. *Alzheimer's Society UK*. Document. 16 February 2021.

https://www.alzheimers.org.uk/sites/default/files/2020-03/communicating_500.pdf

DementiaTalk. 12 July 2017. Document. 19 January 2021.

https://dementiatalk.net/history-of-dementia-when-did-it-all-start/

Draper, Dr Brian. *Dealing With Dementia (A Guide to Alzheimer's Disease and Other Dementias)*. Australia: Allen & Unwin, 2004. Pdf.

https://www.pdfdrive.com/dealing-with-dementia-a-guide-to-alzheimers-disease-and-other-dementias-d156941758.html

Glackin, Partick. *Caring for the Person with Dementia in their Home*. Ireland, April 2013.

G.23.Dementia-Home-Help-Booklet.pdf

MoCA (Montreal Cognitive Assessment). 2019. 28 January 2021.

https://www.mocatest.org/

Phattak, Khrishna Prasad. *An overview on Dementia*. USA: MEDDOCS International, 2018.

https://meddocsonline.org/ebooks/an-overview-on-dementia/an-overview-on-dementia.pdf

"Risk Factors for Dementia." April 2016. *Alzheimer's Society*. 28 January 2021.

https://www.alzheimers.org.uk/sites/default/files/pdf/factsheet_risk_factors_for_dementia.pdf

"Who's Who in Dementia Care." n.d. *NHS*. Document. 16 February 2021.

https://alzheimer.ie/wp-content/uploads/2018/11/A3-Whos-who-in-dementia-care.pdf

We would appreciate it if you could give your precious review of our effort and give your feedback on how we can improve things by writing to us at newbeepublication@gmail.com

or

Visit our website for further publications.

www.newbeepublication.com